MEDICAL PROOFS, SOCIAL EXP.

Medical Proofs, Social Experiments

Clinical Trials in Shifting Contexts

Edited by

CATHERINE WILL
University of Sussex, UK

TIAGO MOREIRA
Durham University, UK

Routledge
Taylor & Francis Group

LONDON AND NEW YORK

First published 2010 by Ashgate Publishing

2 Park Square, Milton Park, Abingdon, Oxon OX14 4RN
711 Third Avenue, New York, NY 10017, USA

Routledge is an imprint of the Taylor & Francis Group, an informa business

First issued in paperback 2016

British Library Cataloguing in Publication Data
Medical proofs, social experiments : clinical trials in
   shifting contexts.
   1. Clinical trials--Social aspects.
   I. Will, Catherine. II. Moreira, Tiago.
   615.5'0724-dc22

Library of Congress Cataloging-in-Publication Data
Medical proofs, social experiments : clinical trials in shifting contexts / [edited] by Catherine Will and Tiago Moreira.
      p. cm.
   Includes bibliographical references and index.
   ISBN 978-0-7546-7928-8 (hardback)
   1. Clinical trials. 2. Drug approval. I. Will, Catherine. II. Moreira, Tiago.
   [DNLM: 1. Clinical Trials as Topic. 2. Drug Approval--methods. QV 771]

   R853.C55M42 2010
   615.5072'4--dc22

                                                          2010030306

ISBN 978-0-7546-7928-8 (hbk)
ISBN 978-1-138-26044-3 (pbk)

Contents

PART III: TESTING THE LIMITS FOR POLICY

List of Contributors

Trudy Dehue: Department of Psychology esp. Principles and History, University of Groningen, Grote Kruisstraat 2/1, 9712 TS Groningen, The Netherlands. Email: g.c.g.dehue@rug.nl.

Alex Faulkner: Centre for Biomedicine & Society, School of Social Science & Public Policy, King's College London, Strand Building (6th Floor), Strand, London, WC2R 2LS. Email: alex.faulkner@kcl.ac.uk.

Ben Heaven: Institute of Health & Society, Newcastle University, Medical Sciences New Build, Richardson Road, Newcastle upon Tyne, NE2 4AX. Email: b.r.j.heaven@ncl.ac.uk.

Claes-Fredrik Helgesson: Department of Thematic Studies – Technology and Social Change, Linköping University, SE-581 83 Linköping, Sweden. Email clae-fredrik.helgesson@liu.se.

Ann Kelly: Anthropologies of African Biosciences Research Group, Health Policy Unit, London School of Hygiene and Tropical Medicine, 15–17 Tavistock Place, London, WC1H 9SH. Email: ann.kelly@lshtm.ac.uk.

Tiago Moreira: School of Applied Social Sciences, Durham University, 32 Old Elvet, Durham, DH1 3HN. Email: tiago.moreira@durham.ac.uk.

Stefan Timmermans: UCLA Department of Sociology, 266 Haines Hall, Los Angeles, CA90095-155, United States. Email: stefan@soc.ucla.edu.

Catherine Will: Department of Sociology, University of Sussex, Friston Building, Falmer, Brighton, BN1 9SP. Email: c.will@sussex.ac.uk.

Introduction
Medical Proofs, Social Experiments:
Clinical Trials in Shifting Contexts

Catherine Will and Tiago Moreira

What kinds of 'work' must be done, and in what locations, to make credible medical proofs? Who and what is involved in the production and articulation of evidence to inform decisions about the organisation and distribution of healthcare in contemporary societies? In this collection we explore the importance and continued evolution of the controlled clinical trial as a key technique for producing evidence in medicine, and for mediating between pharmaceutical companies, clinicians, governments and the public.

In the first half of the 20th century a number of different methodological factors came together to inform new experimental approaches to estimating the effects of treatments, through comparisons between different groups of patients. The use of randomisation to create these comparison groups, and the emphasis on further techniques such as blinding to manage clinical optimism, became increasingly important as trial methodology became standardised as part of efforts to manage the claims made by the pharmaceutical industry (Marks, 1997). Since the institutionalisation, in the 1960s, of the requirement to demonstrate clinical efficacy as well as safety in order to obtain therapeutic marketing licences in the United States and Europe, randomised controlled trials (RCTs) have been an integral part of drug research and development. Indeed the organisation of trials is now a sizeable industry in its own right, consuming many billions of dollars from global pharmaceutical spending on research and development every year.[1]

Increasingly such trials have not only been used to adjudicate on safety or efficacy, but also to help understand the everyday value of treatments *and* set priorities for spending across health care organisations. In this context, there has been an increase in trials designed to assess 'effectiveness', defined as the benefit of an intervention under usual conditions (rather than the 'ideal' conditions produced in a highly controlled efficacy trial). Meanwhile governments have supported a wide range of trials directly, filling in the gaps left by commercial R&D. In the UK since the 1990s these aims have been furthered by the Health

---

1   Global pharmaceutical spending was approximately $55 billion in 2000, 40% of which was dedicated to clinical trials of new drugs (http./ec.europa.eu/internal_market/indprop/docs/invent/patentingdna_en.pdf).

Technology Assessment programme, incorporated into a new National Institute for Health Research in 2007 (which budgeted more than £60 million for trials in its first year).[2] In the US, the economic stimulus package of 2009 included more than $1bn for 'comparative effectiveness research' with the hope of allowing efficiency savings within the growing public healthcare sector.

Yet the greater visibility of trials, their cost, and their importance in the broader politics of healthcare have fed concerns about the accuracy and availability of this evidence base. Commentators suggest that the original purposes of the clinical trial – to provide a fair, robust assessment of the safety, efficacy and effectiveness of a health technology – is being undermined by biased publication and interpretation (Abraham and Lewis, 2000; Dickersin, et al. 1987). This raises issues not only of public trust in regulatory institutions but also of public health, as decisions based on such data can harm individuals and populations. For the purposes of this introduction we describe these concerns in terms of three broad critiques of the RCT and the uses made of it in health care today.[3]

Three Critiques and Some Responses

As the stakes around the use of the clinical trials have been growing, critical voices have multiplied. The diagnoses of the problems with the current organisation of clinical research vary, but here we identify three types of critique: methodological, economic and sociological, before considering some of the responses from within the trials community.

The Methodological Critique

The first critique comes from clinical researchers and statisticians themselves, and proposes that the RCT no longer provides an adequate estimation of the effect of the drug being tested. Such critique proceeds by elaborating on the methodological difficulties of doing trials, and on ways to mitigate their effects using new techniques for data review and summation. Because of the possibilities for bias in the design of trials, and uncertainty arising from interpreting divergent estimations of effect produced by different studies of the same type of intervention, since the late 1980s methodologists have developed a variety of techniques to compile, select and analyse the pooled results of similar studies in systematic reviews and meta-analyses (Eggers, et al. 2001). In a previous paper, Moreira (2007) therefore suggested that the work of systematic reviewers is strongly underpinned by a 'sceptical attitude' towards clinical trial design, management, and reporting. They see clinical trials' reports as rhetorical attempts to convince readers of the value of a drug and their job as reviewers to devise and implement

---

2   http://www.nihr.ac.uk/files/pdfs/NIHR%20Progress%20REport%20200-2008.pdf.

3   Here we draw from Boltanski and Thevenot's (1999) concept of critique.

techniques that neutralise these attempts while recovering valuable data. As results of RCTs are pooled together and tabled, single trials gain a relative meaning where it is possible to reconstruct how researchers' and sponsors' claims differ from the 'overall picture of effect'.

The Economic Critique

The second critique builds on trial data, but proposes incorporating it into further calculations designed to capture the broader value of medical interventions. It suggests that clinical trials, however good they are, do not provide a good enough basis to make decisions about how to produce health in society. For health economists, the production of health is underpinned by an agency relationship whereby the doctor acts on behalf of the patient without usually taking into account the price paid by the patient, insurance company or tax-payer in obtaining or pursuing treatment (e.g. McGuire, Henderson and Mooney, 1986). While clinical trials might be pivotal in offsetting the asymmetry of this relationship by providing health care buyers with an estimation of the clinical gain produced by different treatments, they do not address the question of how to decide on the 'value' of this gain. As Ashmore et al. (1989) have suggested in their analysis of the practices and strategies of health economists during the 1980s, the development of tools to ascertain such value was fraught with controversy as it became intimately linked with emerging debates about health care rationing (Callahan, 1987; Mechanic, 1995).

One of the most successful of these valuation tools was the Quality Adjusted Life Year (QALY), which is denoted by a cost-utility approach that attempts to measure the effects of technologies beyond life expectancy or clinically defined outcomes. In this, the estimation of gain derives from modelling, often based on RCT results, how different scenarios of resource utilisation produce different amount of 'utility,' and what is gained from transferring resources from one scenario to another. Since the 1990s such techniques have been applied in new institutions – of which the UK's National Institute of Health and Clinical Excellence is a prominent example. There, trials are used to inform judgements about the clinical *and* cost effectiveness of drugs as the basis for decisions about whether they will be reimbursed.

The Sociological Critique

Finally what one might call a sociological critique suggests that manufacturers and other interested groups have been able to use the methodological requirements of the RCT to their own advantage, and that over-reliance on trial results therefore skews our understanding of health interventions. Its sociological character derives from seeing the shift in the aims and implementation of the clinical trial as a consequence of the economic and social power exerted by groups in the regulatory process. In some versions, these are seen as subversion or distortions of the experimental form, which can be corrected with stricter adherence to methodological rules, and systems of accountability to police research practices. In many ways, the very strategies of randomisation and double blinding appear early responses to this kind of critique. More recently, Abraham (1995) has suggested that scientists and companies should be held to their own methodological standards to guard against 'bias' in drug regulation.

Other versions of the sociological critique are concerned with understanding how changes in the architecture of clinical trials affect and are affected by the social and political relationships that surround them. For example, a stream of qualitative studies of the everyday organisation of trials have focussed on the ways in which trials build on and further consolidate hierarchical relationships between different professional groups and patients, and have thus identified problems in operation of ethical frameworks centred on the autonomous individual giving 'informed consent' to randomisation and to the use of controls (Featherstone and Donovan, 2002; Corrigan, 2003). Other studies, focussed on the 'political economy of trials' provide stronger critiques of the ways in which trials serve commercial ends (e.g. Rajan, 2006; Sismondo, 2007; Fisher, 2009), and shape the distribution of health. For example Fisher's (2009) analysis of the organisation of clinical research in the US also has some striking similarities with discussions of the ways in which trials become a form of treatment for disadvantaged populations or groups, in Latin America, Eurasia, Africa and Eastern Europe (e.g. Lakoff, 2005; Rajan, 2006; Molyneux and Geissler, 2008; Petryna, 2009).

Responses: The Continued Evolution of the Clinical Trial

The three critiques described above should not be understood as external to the world of clinical research. Proponents of 'Evidence Based Medicine' (EBM) who have been powerful advocates of the trial as the best way to reduce uncertainty about the effects of drugs and other medical interventions have also been at the forefront of research on methodological *and* sociological issues surrounding the use of RCT results. Though EBM began as an effort to get individual doctors to continually challenge the assumptions underlying their practice, it has increasingly had a regulatory face expressed in new technologies such as clinical guidelines or care pathways, which distil trial evidence for everyday use (Berg and Timmermans, 2003). This has been closely tied to the development of techniques for systematic review, and intensified pressure for other improvements to the methodologies surrounding the comparison at the heart of the experimental set up.

A key current concern has been calls for trial registration to reduce the effects of what is known as 'publication bias' where results from negative or equivocal trials do not become publicly available (e.g. Simes, 1986) – a phenomenon with clear risks for systematic reviewers. There has also been growing scrutiny of the choice of endpoints for trials. 'Hard' endpoints such as mortality, or independently measured physiological changes, have been proposed as offering less space than clinical assessments for creative reporting of results. Requiring a commitment to these endpoints across the process of trial design, power calculations and analysis may limit the possibility of 'data dredging' while moves to report trials through absolute rather than relative risk reductions may reduce the ability of manufacturers to inflate their claims for individual products. At the same time new outcomes measures have been derived for concepts such as Quality of Life (Armstrong et al., 2007). These can be presented as giving a closer approximation to patient priorities for treatment, as well as being articulated within economic as well as clinical evaluations. A further discussion has surrounded the nature of trial populations, with a movement to require more diverse groups to be included in trials in order to ensure the broad applicability of results (Epstein, 2007). As well as reducing the potential for commercial bias in trial design and interpretation, new methodological strategies may thus be linked to the desire to make trial results more 'relevant' to real world problems and populations. As the debates about registration, outcomes and inclusion suggest, they also reflect broader interest in transparency, opening up trials to public scrutiny and debate, and there has been much recent interest in the suggestion that researchers should 'involve' the public and patients in their design and in setting research priorities (e.g. Thornton, 2008).

The chapters in this collection explore this evolving picture, in which the ongoing commercialisation of medical research is accompanied by efforts to improve the value of trial research through methodological improvements, regulation and new forms of involvement. Taking both critiques and responses seriously, we explore trials as a powerful stimulus for broader and deeper processes of experimentation in different social and organisational contexts. In doing so, we build on detailed analyses of trials that come out of the field broadly defined as Science and Technology Studies (STS), as a means of exploring the connections that may be made between producing knowledge and producing social orders, or between the emergence of experimentation in science and particular forms of political life (Shapin and Schaffer, 1985; Dear, 2002). In the following sections we introduce a number of themes from previous social scientific analysis of the RCT, before drawing on this literature to elaborate our own theoretical interest in the practices of research and the work required for the interpretation and articulation of medical evidence.

Making Sense of the Political Life of Trials

Regulatory Regimes and Professional Politics

The first starting point for our analysis of the controlled clinical trial is a set of historical studies focussing on the importance of trials for regulation, and their implications for the medical profession. Most prominent is the work of Marks (1997) who suggests that the use of the clinical trial as an instrument of regulation of medical work can be linked to a historical shift in institutional mechanisms of trust, which led reformers to favour what Porter (1995) has named 'mechanical objectivity' in place of personal trust in professionals. A concomitant view grounded in Foucauldian studies of governmentality argues that the rise of the clinical trial is closely connected to the welfare state's demands for efficiency and impersonality (Dehue 2001; 2002; and this volume; Gray and Harrison eds. 2004). For Cambrosio and colleagues (2006) trials are part of emerging 'platforms' which link science and policy in new and significant ways, a phenomenon they characterise as 'regulatory objectivity'. In their account, the control achieved in the experiment may prove to embody a second trial of the ability to regulate, in addition to the effects of treatment.

Though these accounts emphasis the growing authority of the trial, Marks (1997) also acknowledges limitations to this picture. He suggests that trials were part of an 'incomplete revolution' among doctors as statisticians forged alliances with 'therapeutic reformers' around the value of trials, but failed to educate ordinary clinicians about the statistical importance of techniques of sampling and randomisation. Despite legislation mandating the use of trials for drug licensing in the 1960s, this left plenty of space for bitter disagreements about the appropriate design of studies, which he illustrates with several historical cases. Studies of contemporary trials have also emphasised that statistical methods rarely end controversies, and suggest that they rather become the vehicle for conflict between professional groups (Richards, 1991) or coalitions of doctors, scientists and patients (Epstein, 1995; Epstein, 1996; Epstein, 1997; Moreira and Palladino, 2005).

Where does that leave arguments about the contributions of trials to health care policy and regulation? For Berg and Timmermans (2003) the application of a trial protocol is one expression of pressures for standardisation in clinical practice, and an important model or template for instruments such as guidelines, care pathways and even more intricate decision support tools which have the potential to discipline professional work. Yet their empirical studies of these instruments in contrasting areas of US and Netherlands healthcare revealed the local effort and adaptation required to implement a protocol. In these examples professional discretion repeatedly re-emerged, one of many unexpected effects on clinical work. Other research suggests that the emergence of local or national guidelines does not reduce the need for professional discretion, but relocates it to expert leaders or elites (Friedson, 1984; Armstrong, 2002). In the UK Armstrong and Ogden (2006) have also drawn attention to the ongoing importance of individual experimentation in the clinic, irrespective of trial evidence on a particular drug.

On the other hand, May (2006) describes how regulatory agencies may become impatient with the cost (in time and money) of rigorous trials, which do not always match the requirements of policy makers. This is illustrated in work on telemedicine, where May and colleagues find that clinical trials are often rather fragile collaborative endeavours (May and Ellis, 2001). In trials designed to inform policy in this way, the struggle for *relevance* means researchers have to come to terms with the institutional setting and accommodate variation between practitioners and patients (Will, 2007). Such processes of 'contextualisation' or 'epistemic emplacement' (Street, undated) complicate the links made between trials and public health across different national and local contexts – an important factor given the continued internationalisation of clinical research activity.

The Publics of Health Research

As the trial industry has expanded and travelled, a rich literature has emerged on the ways in which trials intersect with the pursuit of 'public health' at local and national levels. Epstein's (1996) work on the priorities and design of AIDS research in the 1980s has become a classic – describing a case where patients rushed to access trials as a source of treatment, but also demanded new approaches to their design to hasten results and distribute potential benefits. Other cases in the Euro-American context also reveal the ways in which designing and carrying out trials may become part of a much broader social negotiation of medical innovation, for example in genetics (Rabeharisoa and Callon, 2002) or regenerative medicine (Moreira and Palladino, 2005), where patient groups may ally with researchers to produce visions of effective treatment and make claims on public funding for further trials.

The relationship between research and the provision of healthcare – and therefore public stakes in trials – becomes still more complicated when viewed on a global scale. For example Rajan (2006) draws attention to intense inequality between 'experimental subjects' in India and 'sovereign consumers' of drugs in the US. As Petryna (2009) describes, commercial research organisations working on contract to pharmaceutical companies are engaged in a 'global search for subjects' who are willing to take part in trials. They are increasingly attracted to Eastern Europe, Eurasia and South America, where populations are not taking large numbers of alternative drugs (in comparison with the 'treatment saturation' of populations in the north and west), and where companies are able to build relationships with relatively resource poor clinicians. In addition to feeding off inequity, this enrolment of local clinicians can lead to publicly-funded healthcare (when it is available) being distorted by the use of expensive drugs, or by the extension of diagnostic categories promulgated through new research (e.g. Lakoff, 2005; Petryna, 2009).

Concern with these issues informs calls for new types of ethical discussion, built on investigations of the institutional, national and international contexts of research (e.g. Molyneux and Geissler, 2008). This is intended to supplement ethical frameworks that focus on the individual, and explore the implications of international ethical guidelines as they are applied to very different local and national settings. Using ethnographic work in Poland and Brazil, Petryna (2009) foregrounds the ways in which commercial research operates in the gap between actual healthcare provision and potential benefits. Though such questions have been addressed in international guidelines such as the Helsinki Declaration (first issued in 1964, and repeatedly updated) or in the recent Good Clinical Practice guidelines (from the International Conference on Harmonisation) she argues that researchers actually operate through and with forms of what she calls 'ethical variability', which take account of variations in the standard of care. Effective regulation of trials relies on work by national governments, which must balance clinical ethics against economic, scientific and regulatory constraints and demands. In this context the 'goods' that might result from trials all too often remain private, for though public health providers may become part of the commercial research enterprise, the distribution of the benefits remains uncertain.

A rich vein of work on clinical research therefore continues to raise questions about the effects of trials, beyond their ability to act as straightforward channels for state regulation, or expressions of corporate agendas. Instead we have a picture of diverse and complex negotiations between professionals and patients, governments and industry in different times and places. In this collection we wish to extend this insight, drawing on ethnographic studies of clinical trials in Europe and America to complement the work described above. In particular many of the cases described here come from countries that have a functioning public health care system, contrasting with both the United States and more impoverished settings, where trials appear as a means of accessing care. Furthermore, our ambition to account for the links between research and policy in these contexts is informed by theory developed in relation to other scientific activity, which suggests that experimentation in this broader sense should be seen as a potential form of politics in contemporary societies – with implications that go beyond the tensions and accommodations between health care payers, professionals and patients. This approach is elaborated in our next section, before we summarise the contributions and key themes for the collection as a whole.

Trials as Collective Experiments

The authors of our chapters share an interest in the distributed nature of knowledge production and the unpredictability inherent in experimental work even in the relatively regulated and standardised form of the randomised controlled clinical trial. In a strict sense, the experiment is a scientific practice that aims to 'test' a particular proposition/hypothesis. However, the history of experimentalism has demonstrated that from the 17th century onwards experiments have also offered ways of organising and mediating social and political relations, or bringing to bear the concerns of the polity (Schaffer, 2005). Thus philosopher Isabelle Stengers (2000) has argued that the traditional view of experiments is an impoverished version of the process of experimentation, which she conceptualises as an 'event' in that it is able to generate new and 'interesting' entities for the actors – human and non-human – engaged in its production, and new connections between human affairs and the management and production of things. Though the clinical trial may be presented by scientists and policy makers as a machine to produce facts through the hypothetico-deductive model, or an experiment in its narrow definition, the political importance of trials leads us to consider them as experimentation in this broader sense. Indeed, for Latour (2004), this richer view of experimental work is critical for responses to the most pressing issues in technological societies, which frequently face multi-layered uncertainty.

> When it is no longer possible to define a single nature and multiple cultures, the collective has to explore the question of the number of entities to be taken into account and integrated [...] From the 'experimentation', as it is used in the sciences, I borrow the following: it is instrument-based, rare, difficult to reproduce, always contested and it presents itself as a costly trial whose result has to be decoded (ibid.: 238).

While this is framed as a normative suggestion, others have suggested that such practices of collective experimentation are already in use in certain domains. Callon, for example, has argued that processes such as the involvement of patient associations in health research, are already part of a new regime of knowledge production (Callon, 2004; Callon, Lascoumes and Barthe, 2001; Rabeharisoa and Callon, 2002). He suggests the characteristics of this regime – open membership, open-endedness, distributedness – are also evident across more traditional forms of knowledge production. Our suggestion is that contemporary clinical trials may also display such characteristics, as the experimental method is applied to diverse settings and subject to increased scrutiny and debate. Thus the chapters in this book investigate the ways in which the work of research is distributed between different actors, and across time and space; and how debates about the design, organisation, interpretation and evaluation of a clinical trial extend beyond the clinical research community to different collectives.

We noted above that cases of passionate patient involvement in trials described by Epstein (1996) and Rabeharisoa and Callon (2002) have been used as exemplars of a more general shift in the dynamics of knowledge production (Irwin and Michael, 2003; Latour, 1998). For some of our authors this is also linked to the idea of science explicitly produced for and interwoven with the needs of society – what Gibbons (1999) describes as Mode 2 knowledge. In this model, new dynamic collaborations are emerging between the institutions of industry, state and academia, *and* an informed public. If patient activism serves here to illustrate the political power of public involvement, our contributors further open up questions about the meaning of 'involvement' in different registers, including individual patients, health care professionals, citizens and wider publics.

Furthermore, such involvement is expressed and demanded through broader institutional innovation and the ongoing 'reflexive management' of scientific work (Nowotny et al. 2001). Even 'traditional' trials therefore require complex negotiations about the resources that can be marshalled to put into the experiment, and the distribution of goods that may come out. Pressures for relevance, transparency and accountability require new forms of work as part of research. New institutions are being called into being to produce more subtle, distributed and visible evaluations of trial results.

This collection offers a series of empirical, and therefore carefully located, investigations of these developments in the significance of the RCT, animated by questions about the kinds of 'work' that are involved in carrying out a trial and producing credible data. What relationships, goods and values are invoked and produced by the design and organisation of different clinical trials? How have the results of such studies been incorporated in wider social, political and technical debates about contemporary health care? And can the clinical trial be re-designed or re-imagined to satisfy social and political expectations introduced by appeals to evidence-based or informed policy?

Studying Trials in Practice

In seeking to answer these questions and others like them, social scientists working in a qualitative tradition face interesting challenges, as they come into contact with people who claim particular authority for both quantitative data and the experimental approach. Though they locate themselves in different disciplines (history, sociology, philosophy, anthropology), the authors in this collection each bring close empirical work to answer our questions, in contrast to a number of commentaries produced from ethics or the philosophy of science, which to some extent are reliant on formal claims made about clinical trials rather than their actual, and diverse, instantiation (Norheim, 2002; Worrall, 2002; Ashcroft and Meulen, 2004; Cartwright, 2007). Many of our chapters are ethnographic in a broad sense, coming out of sustained engagement with particular locations, groups or organisations. This ethnographic perspective provides a space to explore the complex and contingent resolutions of the debates that follow trials, probing the investments of different collectives in particular forms of evaluation, and the ways in which scientific and social decisions are co-produced in situations of interpretative flexibility left by the clinical trial. Here the work of doing trials, or 'research', is not imagined as somehow distinct from clinical work, or 'practice', but rather the two are seen to evolve or emerge together, with sometimes unexpected outcomes for science, for medicine and for policy. The book therefore provides ways to think about the continued development of the clinical trial, and consider how it might meet the challenges of new technologies and health care costs in the future, through discussions of three broad areas: a) the practices of research; b) collective efforts at their interpretation; and c) the use of trials for policy making.

The Practices of Research

The first section is focussed on the practices of research, bringing together ethnographic studies of trials of very different interventions (counselling, professional education and pharmaceuticals), which nevertheless share a number of epistemic and organisational problems. Here the formal presentation of the trial, through a protocol or other forms of documentation, hides different forms of 'work' essential to its operation: work of caring, enrolling staff and participants, and cleaning and verifying data. While the trial protocol therefore inevitably contains one version of clinical practice, these accounts reveal varied, sometimes competing, narratives about the roles played by patients, nurses, doctors and pharmaceutical companies. Thus Timmermans (this volume) offers an example of a trial in which ethical and organisational demands led it to produce a kind of care – what he terms a 'therapeutic haven' – for a desperate and under-served population of drug users. Though the trial appears as a failure if the researchers hoped to provide evidence of the effectiveness of a pharmaceutical to help end addiction, in fact they live with it as a kind of success. In contrast, Heaven (this volume) describes a pilot study that is more widely seen as failure, as efforts to intervene in and discipline professional work produce little change in clinical relationships. Yet the negotiations between these groups, and efforts to bridge what he calls an 'ontological divide' between researchers and practitioners, also reveal the ways in which researchers must work with knowledge about practice, and practitioners produce alternative accounts of experimental behaviour in clinical relationships. The final piece in this section (Helgesson this volume) again addresses the complex connections between research and practice, in a study of the effort that goes into producing information for the pharmaceutical sponsors of large trials. Here pressures for robust and clean data require new forms of work in the clinic, checking records, flagging problems, and then erasing the signs of this work to prepare the data to travel.

Framing Collective Interpretation

The second section builds on accounts of research in practice to consider how attempts to interpret and act on trial results require subsequent efforts to recover the context of data production, and give authority to different accounts of the trial in public. Thus Will (this volume) explores tentative steps to open out and examine the 'collective work' of interpreting trial data through professional exchanges contained in the journal literature. Where Helgesson's chapter reveals practices by research organisations to erase traces of the situations in which data is produced, Will shows how journals attempt to partially reconstruct these situations, and thereby the subtle meanings of the headline results of trials, through particular editorial interventions. For journal editors, trials, though authoritative, form only part of a wider universe of scientific understanding, and other forms of knowledge must be brought to bear in interpreting them. While expert clinicians continue to have an important role in this, efforts are also made to open up the pages of journals to diverse practitioners, and to complete Marks' (1997) incomplete revolution by educating the individual doctor.

In Moreira (this volume) these varied forms of knowledge were more explicitly and extensively debated, as a public controversy about the organisation and funding of Alzheimer's care in the UK sparked efforts to present and contest the economic critique of trials. Again, professional discretion is reasserted, this time with reference to trials as measures of clinical rather than cost effectiveness, but in this case such clinical discretion was somewhat paradoxically accompanied by professional defence of 'mechanical' objectivity tied to trials, set against health economists' attempt to proceed through more reflexive exploration of uncertainty and more pragmatic connections between research and practice.

Testing the Limits for Policy

Our final section continues to explore the unexpected outcomes, and the complex productions, of trials, focussing on the connections drawn between clinical research and public policy in very diverse settings: Dutch psychiatry; international efforts to control malaria; and debates about both osteoporosis and cancer screening in the UK. Here we see attempts to re-imagine trial methodology to manage the weight of expectations from policy makers and patients, but also cases where criticism was ignored and side-lined. For both Dehue and Faulkner, trials have become 'normal science' in assessments of evidence to inform health policy. Dehue (this volume) argues that the reliance on narrow comparisons of pharmaceutical drugs leads to impoverished accounts of therapy for depression in national guidelines.

Kelly (this volume) turns to a case in which trials are applied to cheaper and more prosaic technologies in an effort to produce pragmatic evidence of 'the[ir] effectiveness in the field of everyday practice': here UK general practice, and malaria control in the Gambia. Here social robustness inheres in the way in which notions of 'public good' are central to the design and organisation of trials – but their importance for policy appears heavily contingent on institutional arrangements and funding. Likewise, Faulkner (this volume) describes a case where trials repeatedly failed to provide answers that were given weight in policy. In this case researchers entered into a more prolonged and self-conscious reinvention of the trial format incorporating qualitative research to produce versions of patient beliefs, expectations and perspectives to feed into its design. As in Dehue's critical account (this volume) this remained somewhat individualising in its emphasis, but strikingly it asked patients, doctors *and* policy makers to confront areas of uncertainty, rather than allow the controlled comparison to stand for certainty in the contested field of screening technologies.

The diversity of our cases, representing the use of trials to investigate service innovations as well as pharmaceuticals, different clinical areas (neurology, oncology, cardiology and psychiatry, among others), and different countries (United States, United Kingdom, Netherlands, Sweden and the Gambia) helps give weight to our conclusions about the social as well as clinical experimentation already underway. Much has been written about the attractions of Evidence Based Medicine for policy makers anxious to control the costs of health care with reference to the authority of science. Indeed we increasingly see the rhetoric of 'Evidence Based Policy-Making' applied, or perhaps re-introduced, to other policy areas including crime and justice education and development. Yet even a small set of cases from the field of health care reveals some of the challenges of this approach.

While the RCT may be re-imagined and reanimated to deal with the weight of growing expectations, its value for policy cannot be assumed, and its relationship to clinical care is often complicated. Practice is not a prior given, to which trial results can be applied at the end of the experiment. Rather practice evolves alongside and through efforts at research. In setting up trials, researchers recognise and invoke key collectives – not just patients, but also diverse professional groups, policy-makers, and publics. Trials must both operate on and hold in balance different concerns. In attempting to accommodate these, and demands for more general transparency, trials themselves become part of broader forms of experimentation. While we would not wish to disagree with Petryna's (2009) arguments about the importance of commercial actors in shaping this exploration, local groups (patients/professionals) and national actors (governments, regulatory institutions) are also relevant. Here notions of public involvement and public good must be carefully interrogated, and not only through an ethical lens.

Finally, our chapters testify to the fact that the RCT is not a static institution itself, but a subject for ongoing work by methodologists and clinical researchers, who attempt to respond to criticisms of the RCT even as they defend its ability to reduce uncertainty. We might add to these 'internal' efforts at critique and reform a concern with those contextual factors that shape what a trial can do. Issues such as mobilising and retaining participants, locating funding, choosing comparators and assigning professional roles are not incidental to the assessment of efficacy or effectiveness that is the ideal result of a trial. Indeed such difficulties might be seen as critical to any understanding of the value of the experiment, and how its results might be incorporated into regulation or changes to professional practice. A key challenge then is finding ways to talk about and acknowledge the difficulties of producing credible evidence, and ways to get trials to carry information about their conditions of production away from the research site, and into journals, policy documents, guidelines and consulting rooms.

PART I
The Practices of Research

The chapters in this section deal with the challenges attendant on the production of evidence using trial methodology. In so doing, they complicate notions of success or failure in relation to such research. The challenges are many: the nature of both experimental intervention and 'control' must be agreed; professional work should be aligned with the requirements of the experiment; data must be collected, corrected and verified; outcomes agreed and measured; and convincing accounts prepared of the work of the trial and its meaning. It is common, in some critiques of trials, to contrast 'research' with 'practice' where one is dry and rigid, while the other is peopled and flexible. Here the practices of research emerge as just as complex as those of everyday clinical work, animated no less by professional rivalries or ambitions, including the urge to provide care, and reliant on local efforts to come to fruition.

The first two chapters offer ethnographic accounts of individual trials that deal with 'research' as a disruption to clinical practice; either overlaying new services on a gap in provision for a neglected group (Timmermans) or attempting to get clinical staff to try new approaches to a common clinical problem (Heaven). In the first case, health care professionals construe the trial as an opportunity to provide care to people dependent on methamphetamine in the US, despite the lack of efficacy demonstrated for the pharmaceutical treatment of its intervention arm. In the second, UK-based practitioners resist research into behavioural interventions with patients as a distraction from ongoing primary care. Despite these differences the research effort in each case looks very similar. In both, worries about recruitment and retention lead the trial team to do a great deal of what Heaven terms 'hidden work' to make their intervention, and the trial as a whole, acceptable for patients and professionals, and thus to successfully enroll them in the research endeavour. This requires changing behaviour and accepting interventions to account for those changes through measurements of different outcomes.

In the third chapter, the hidden work is that of data cleaning, as Helgesson describes the different layers of checking that go into the preparation of a dataset before large multi-centre drug trials, funded by pharmaceutical companies, can be unblinded. Again much of this work is local, indeed it should be local. As Helgesson notes, research nurses, investigators and monitors engage in textual practices at the trial sites to repair, or tidy up, inconsistencies or absences in the records, and subsequently to make traces of this work 'disappear'. At the same time, staff at data management organisations are suspicious of data that appears too 'clean' upon arrival: perfect data is a sign of fraud, and 'data that is clean by itself is the dirtiest data of all.' Helgesson's chapter brings to the fore how mundane judgements about the organisation and appearance of 'raw data' work to secure the quality of the data produced by trials.

In each case then, the practices of research mix efforts to achieve abstraction at the point of outcomes with local work to implement the protocol, work which is necessarily imbued with the collective politics of each site, not least tensions between doctors, nurses, and other professionals. Our contributors describe many different efforts to manage such tensions, and discipline practice, including telling stories about times when things went wrong: Heaven's 'atrocity stories' and Helgesson's 'cautionary tales'. Yet in each case researchers also acknowledge the importance of finding more positive ways to 'involve' staff and patients, illustrated even in the example presented by Heaven, as the appeal to work in an 'experimental mode' offers another way to include staff in the search for new knowledge and understanding.

Chapter 1

Reconciling Research with Medical Care in RCTs

Stefan Timmermans

In *Experiment Perilous* (1959), pioneering medical sociologist Renée Fox studied physicians and patients in a metabolic research hospital unit participating in an emerging practice in biomedicine: the mixture of clinical care with medical research. Observing clinicians experimenting with last-resort medical interventions, Fox noted first-hand what is still a vexing problem in clinical research: how to weigh the broader epistemic pay-off for aggregate patient populations against the direct benefits of participation in research as a form of care for individual patients. Her analysis of the staff centred upon uncertainties stemming from the dual role of researcher and clinician and coping mechanisms for dealing with these uncertainties. She explained:

> As clinical investigators, [the physicians] were not only obligated to protect and further the welfare of their patients, but they were also responsible for advancing general medical knowledge. Thus, their decisions about whether or not they ought to undertake a certain measure generally involved a rather complicated moral titration process. In some cases they had to balance the potential risks of the technique or agent they wished to test against its presumed significance for the welfare of the patients who acted as subjects and for the furtherance of knowledge. In other cases, where the patients on whom it was tried could not expect to be helped by it, they had to weigh the possible contribution such an experimental procedure or drug might make to medical science and the 'good of society' in general against the suffering and hazards it might involve for these patients (Fox, 1959: 241).

In this early medical sociological work about biomedical research, the central issue was thus the reconciliation of the competing demands between taking care of individual patients and producing generalizable scientific knowledge. While sometimes these two goals coincided, more often specific interventions may not benefit individual patients but be performed solely for their research value. Or alternatively, individual care demands may invalidate broader research aims.

Fox wrote at a time of great clinical autonomy in balancing research and patient care in which the boundary of acceptable experimental interventions was determined by the research staff. In the aftermath of well-known transgressions in which researchers took advantage of vulnerable populations to conduct biomedical research, concern about balancing generalisable knowledge with the care needs of individual patients in biomedical trials has led to a series of regulatory interventions. Sydney Halpern (2004) distinguishes three phases of social control in the US: the first phase goes back to the 18th century and runs to the early decades of the 20th century and consists of *informal control* of communities of scientists who embraced a logic of lesser harms. A potentially hazardous clinical intervention was acceptable if it yielded net benefits and its risks were lower than natural disease. The second period runs until the 1960s. During that time, organisations sponsoring medical research required *oversight procedures* for managing the risks of clinical experiments, including written informed consent procedures and insurance for scientists. In the third phase, when accounts of gross research misconduct were published, government organisations began to formally *regulate* human experimentation. This is the advent of institutionalised review boards (IRB) adopting an autonomy-based approach to managing research risks and benefits and requiring voluntary research participation and informed consent of subjects. Currently, all research involving human subjects in the US that receives federal funding or involves federal agencies requires IRB approval.

The bureaucratisation of research going back at least to the 1960s in the US has not resolved the tension of combining individual patient care and research aims.

Bioethicists continue to warn against the danger of patients overestimating benefits of participating in clinical trials (the 'therapeutic misconception,' see (Kimmelman, 2007)) and against the risks of procedures that have mainly research purposes (Miller and Rosentstein, 2003). At the same time, policy makers have argued for more equitable access to potentially life-saving clinical trials (Epstein, 1996, 2007), arguing that trial participation is a scarce social good that needs to be distributed equitably. In addition, some observers have argued that clinical trials have increasingly begun to serve a residual health care function in a country such as the US with ingrained health care inequities (Fisher, 2009; Timmermans and McKay, 2009), similar to the ways that clinical trials are marketed in countries with crumbling health infrastructures (Petryna, 2009). As a result, sociologists and anthropologists have documented how trials perpetuate inequities in the US (Fox, 1959; Fishman, 2004; Orr, 2006) and around the globe (Abraham, 1995, 2007; Rajan, 2003; Lakoff, 2005; Petryna, 2006; Heimer, 2007) by exposing desperate populations to ill-understood risks (Lidz, Appelbaum, Grisso and Renaud, 2004). Social scientists (Mirowski and Van Horn, 2005; Sismondo, 2008; Fisher, 2009) and increasingly medical observers (Shuchman, 2007), have also warned about the changing landscape of new corporate-sponsored clinical research infrastructures and gaps in regulatory oversight.

While the risks are well-covered in the social science literature and the strengths and weaknesses of the knowledge gained from trials have been parsed out in great detail, we know little of how within such a regulated environment research staff and participants within clinical trials reconcile the mixture of care with research (see also Kelly and Faulkner, this volume). Relying on observations and in-depth interviews with participants and staff of a trial testing a pharmaceutical for methamphetamine dependency, I will review how these parties aim to simultaneously achieve treatment in a research setting and conduct research to gain broader efficacious treatment knowledge. I will show that the combination of research and treatment as framed by regulatory demands creates tensions between care and experimentation but also has some unexpected results. Specifically, the provision of treatment in a research setting, especially for a condition for which few alternative treatments are available, generates an attractive treatment environment that is confidential, free of cost, and staffed with caring and medically trained experts, a situation intensified by the requirement to have therapies available for participants in the placebo arm. A randomised clinical trial that does not show statistically significant pharmacological efficacy can thus still have beneficial treatment benefits for some individual participants.

Methodology

The data for this chapter is drawn from an observational study of a randomised clinical trial for methamphetamine dependency. The trial tested bupropion, a norepinephrine and dopamine reuptake inhibitor that has been approved by the FDA as an antidepressant and as a smoking cessation drug. The inclusion criteria of the trial specified that participants needed to be at least 18 years old, met the DSM criteria for methamphetamine dependency, and consented to the study procedures. Besides bupropion or a placebo, the trial required thrice weekly urine samples for a 12-week period, and offered an opportunity for cognitive-behavioural therapy, and contingency management. The staff also collected various batteries of cognitive tests and outcome data. The trial aimed for 70 research subjects in two research sites.

I observed and interviewed the staff and trial participants over a one-year period, conducting interviews with 10 staff members and 40 participants. This interview data was analyzed in a modified grounded theory-analytical induction approach where data suggested emerging analytical themes against a close reading of the social scientific and medical literature (Timmermans and Tavory, 2007).

Methamphetamine Dependency

Metamphetamine has been used in medicine for eighty years but the legitimate indications are now limited. The drug is currently mainly prescribed as a short-term appetite suppressant or narcopletic agent and occasionally as a treatment for hyper-activity disorder. The DEA has classified the drug as a Schedule II substance meaning that it is a drug with some legitimate indications but a high potential for abuse and dependency. Methamphetamine remains an easily available and widely used psychostimulant among all sections of the population, but particularly among blue-collar workers, college students and in gay/lesbian communities. Compared to cocaine, methamphetamine has a prolonged half-life and duration of action. Methamphetamine enters the brain and triggers a release of dopamine, norephinephrine and serotonin causing almost instantaneous feelings of excitement when the drug is smoked, snorted, drunk, or injected. Methamphetamine is addictive and prolonged use may lead to paranoia and delusions, hypertension, heart damage, strokes and deteriorating dental health. Quitting methamphetamine may lead to withdrawal symptoms such as drug cravings, depression, and excessive sleeping.

In 2006, the US had an estimated 731,000 users of methamphetamine (SAMHSA, 2007), but they had few treatment options (Winslow, Voorhees, and Pehl, 2007); most of those who quit seem to do it on their own (Borders, Booth, Han, Wright, Leukefeld, Falck et al., 2008). Review articles of methamphetamine treatments indicate that 'there are no evidence-based practices that have been developed specifically for the treatment of methamphetamine use disorders' (Roll, 2007: 114). In particular, research on pharmaceutical treatments remains in its infancy (Elkashef, Rawson, Smith, Pearce, Flammino, Campbell et al., 2007). People looking for treatment can access peer-support groups such as Narcotics Anonymous, court-mandated treatments, and – in rare instances – in-patient treatments. Generally, a treatment gap remains between supply and demand for methamphetamine dependency (Wright, Sathe, and Spagnola, 2007). Nationally in 2006, 7.8 million people needed treatment for drug addiction but only 1.6 million or 20% received treatment. Among the reasons for not receiving treatment were lack of insurance, not knowing where to go for treatment, concern about stigma or negative repercussions at work and in the community, and not ready to quit using (SAMHSA, 2007). Participants in the clinical trial confirmed the lack of treatment options: few had experience with in-patient or out-patient rehabilitation services. Besides trying to quit on their own, they had mainly relied on voluntary, peer-support groups, which the physician involved in the study referred to as 'necessary but not sufficient' for recovery.

The randomised, double-blind, placebo-controlled trial offered a comprehensive set of free and confidential treatment components. The trial staff presented the pharmaceuticals tested in the trial not as cures but as tools to take the edge off methamphetamine cravings and withdrawal symptoms. A physician administered the medications and also conducted a physical examination, including EKGs and an HIV test, to determine eligibility for the trial and monitor any adverse reactions. Regulatory agencies mandate that every participant should receive tangible benefits from participating in the trial. Because half the trial population would receive a placebo, the entire trial population was invited to participate in individual counselling sessions in cognitive-behavioural therapy consisting of interventions that attempt to foster abstinence by increasing skills for coping with high-risk situations. During the sessions, the counsellors provided weekly tasks to focus on self-monitoring and relapse analysis, identification of 'triggers' and cognitive and/or behavioural strategies for coping with them, problem-solving skills, education about methamphetamine and methamphetamine dependence, education about HIV and reducing the risk of HIV transmission, and motivation/ commitment to stopping drug use.

To record the outcomes of the trial, the staff requested that the participants provide three urine samples (Monday, Wednesday and Friday). The samples were tied to another behavioural intervention, contingency management, where participants were paid for clean samples allowing them to earn a total of $537 over the course of the twelve weeks. Participants started at $3 and for every clean sample they receive an extra dollar until week 4, when the amount stayed at $15. If the urine sample contained methamphetamine traces, the voucher went back to $3. After three clean samples, it returned to the highest value before the dirty sample. Research indicates that contingency management has shown success in both initiating and maintaining periods of abstinence in methamphetamine treatment (Roll, 2007).

While half of the trial population thus received a pharmaceutical, the entire group had the option to participate in a health check-up, cognitive-behavioural therapy and contingency management. In the next section, I first examine how research goals are achieved in a clinical setting, followed by a section on obtaining treatment in a research context. I am particularly interested in the intended and unintended consequences of pursuing both research and therapeutics goals.

Research in a Treatment Setting

On a daily basis, the staff was preoccupied with recruiting participants, gathering and documenting data points, and retaining participants. Retention was a particular challenge as the trial manager explained:

> I've worked on behavior trials and medication trials with methamphetamine and opiate addicts. This is probably the worst follow up I've seen across the studies. People just fall of the face of the planet and really, especially out here, they go to jail or they go off to Texas or something. Everybody just kind of goes off in different directions, so follow up is hard. They're not motivated by the money. The 15 dollars voucher is really not bringing them back.

The staff was faced with further constraints due to strenuous research eligibility requirements. Recruitment for research purposes, for example, was slowed down by extensive psychological and physical screenings and repeated cognitive measures. In addition, conducting the trial in an out-patient clinic meant weighing off increased external validity against problems for data collection. The research staff noted that the conditions of testing drug users while they continued daily life mimicked the typical situation of patients seeking care in a clinic or physician's office. Yet, this greater external validity also made it easier for participants to fail to show up or drop out. The consequence was missing data, not necessarily on the primary outcome data of urine tests but on additional measures. 'Some of the other stuff that you need to parse out why it didn't work, lots of times there is missing data, or just not even missing but a limit to the amount of data.' Commenting on the cumbersome cognitive measures that were collected at different points throughout the study, the physician involved in the study explained: 'particularly some meth-addicted young person doesn't want to sit there for an hour on a computer doing a brain teaser but you need them to do that.'

At the same time, from a purely research perspective, even more stringent eligibility criteria could favourably shape the results of the study. The staff was aware that pharmaceutical companies seemed to be doing better at retaining trial subjects and more likely to produce positive results. They explained these differences in terms of the industry's ability to be more selective in trial screening and offer higher financial incentives. Many research participants were attracted to the study because the trial was free and they would not need to drop out of work and family as required in an in-patient setting. At the same time, the research staff postulated that an in-patient clinic would select for a study population that was more homogeneous and more likely to react positively to the medication: 'So we were just bouncing around ideas like, well, maybe we should put those people in the hospital for five days and just give them some sleeping pills till they wake up clean, let them start getting some of the vouchers and then let them go in the outpatient and take the meds.'

If the goal of the clinical trial set-up was to create the best-possible situation to produce a therapeutic effect of the pharmaceutical being tested, then the researchers would not have offered any alternative treatments. Yet, requirement to offer something to all participants led to the inclusion of psycho-behavioural therapies: 'the counseling and the contingency management make it justifiable to use the placebo. Both of these two things have been shown to help people stop using meth on their own. So we can say we're still giving people the standard of treatment even if they're getting a placebo medication.' The psycho-behavioural therapies combined with the placebo effect provided a positive response rate in the placebo group that the pharmaceutical arm had to significantly surpass for the drug to be counted as effective. In depression studies, the placebo effect alone can account for 50–70% success rate, creating a tremendous hurdle for active medication to overcome (Lakoff, 2007).

Research participants rarely commented on the research purposes of the trial – positively or negatively – except with vague statements that they hoped that their participation would help other users. They were preoccupied with the immediate goal of finding a solution for their own methamphetamine use. The biggest gripe was that staff could not tell them whether they would be receiving the active medication or a placebo. Because the pharmaceutical company had little interest in tapping the methamphetamine market, the company was unwilling to provide the pill and a similar looking placebo. The researchers also could not grind up the medication because that might affect the pharmacological qualities. They thus had to use medication bought in stores. To blind the pill, it was inserted in a large capsule with an equivalent looking capsule for placebo. Trial participants who opened the capsule, as at least one did, would find a pill stamped with 'wellbutrin' and know that they received active medication. Another found out that she received placebo when she swallowed a handful of capsules and did not notice any reaction. Some participants had already taken bupropion as a smoking cessation drug and they had low hopes for the drug's ability to help it with methamphetamine. Yet, the overwhelming sentiment among participants was that they were willing to try something, even research, since nothing else had helped in the past.

Three further characteristics of the trial as a research endeavour were especially attractive to participants: confidentiality, free treatment, and friendly staff. The trial advertised in print and radio media, encouraging people wanting to quit methamphetamine to call a number. The staff responding to the phone observed that they were asked about 'confidentiality over and over again.' In interviews, trial participants also emphasised that confidentiality was key to their participation. About a quarter of the respondents had health insurance and more had regular access to a physician but few participants approached their health care provider to find out about meth. treatments. At the same time, participants could opt to selectively disclose their participation in a clinical trial to certain people. Participants remained thus in control of who knew about their participation.

Second, a distinguishing characteristic of the treatment was that it was not only free of cost to the participants who may otherwise had to pay several thousand dollars for in-patient treatments, but they also had an opportunity to earn vouchers for groceries, food, and gas. If the trial did not work out, the participant had thus not invested scarce financial resources: 'My kids wanted to send me to this place, all these places. They're so expensive. Well, they were like 10,000 dollars a month, some of them were. You know, and in the back of my head thinking, yeah, if it doesn't work, then I'm really going to hear about the money they spent and whatever. So that's why I didn't want any part of that.' Besides treatment provided through the court system, this was the only treatment available free of cost.

Third, the staff was very motivated to keep the participants enrolled in the trial and tried to reach out to them by being friendly and non-judgmental. The psychologist explained: 'The fact that we're not judging them and making them feel bad is huge.' Participants concurred: 'When I saw [the trial physician], he was, "Don't give up," you know, like "You're doing a good job," or "You need to surprise yourself. You know, you are doing a good job."' This message was reinforced by all staff members: 'I was looking forward every three days to coming here, you know, because I needed to quit and these guys were so positive about everything. The doc and [site manager] and [study director] and everybody here. I wasn't clean for the first four weeks. I was still using and my samples were still dirty and stuff. And they were so encouraging about it. They were, you know, like, "Come on, man! You've got to finish it."' While staff members were careful not to become personally involved in the participants' life situation, they rooted for continuation in the trial. This personalised approach could still affect research participation: 'Some people do end up dropping or stop coming because they almost feel like they let us down.' To avoid losing participants this way, the case worker told participants: 'It's great that you're ... you're getting yourself clean. Don't ever feel like you can't come here, you know, if you're not clean.'

In sum, the research staff was occupied with recruitment, retention and obtaining the necessary data points for analysis but participants were largely unconcerned about these specific research activities, focusing instead on the particulars of the RCT routine and their goal of becoming drug free. Participants interpreted encouragement to finish the trial regardless of clean urine samples as staff taking a personal interest in their wellbeing. Some participants expressed frustration with not knowing whether they received active or placebo medication. Regulatory protection of human research subjects in biomedical research, as well as limited resources, may have created additional barriers by confounding pharmacological effects with proven psycho-behavioural treatments and by limiting recruitment selectivity. The trial's external validity was high but this clinical realism may have actually rendered it more difficult to prove drug efficacy.

Receiving Treatment in a Research Environment

While meeting research aims of recruitment, data points, and retention was a salient concern for the staff, obtaining effective treatment was relevant to both staff and participants. Research results were not available until after the study was unblinded but ongoing interactions between staff and participants were framed by addressing drug dependency. As mentioned above, alternative treatments for methamphetamine use were either mandated by courts, expensive and therefore unavailable, or based on peer-support with little accountability. In contrast, the clinical trial offered a variety of treatment options including medical supervision, individual counselling, contingency management, and the pharmaceutical being tested. While not everyone appreciated all options, most participants found something to their liking.

Because of the secretive nature of drug use, few participants had confided their addiction to primary health care providers. In fact, when asked whether he had talked to his HIV physician about meth, a participant echoing others replied 'why in the hell would you want to do that? Once they see you as a drug addict, they always see you as a drug addict.' Therefore, the opportunity to talk to a physician was appreciated across the sample: 'it was nice to finally be able to tell a doctor really what was going on. Because I can't tell my regular doctor,' cause, you know how they are. I mean, I remember when I was having the baby. I didn't get any prenatal care, partially because fucking ... I didn't want them to pick up on the fact that I was on meth.'

The physician in the study conducted a physical examination, monitored the participants for adverse effects, and answered questions about treatment modalities. Because many participants had not accessed a physician in years, he addressed issues related to delayed care, even diagnosing several patients with chronic conditions and referring them to other care providers for follow-up care. Several participants also valued the close monitoring of drug withdrawal: 'I wanted to be monitored by a doctor. Because I really think that you need to be monitored because, you quit doing dope, your arteries open back up. Your heart's pumping a lot of blood slowly.'

The physician's contributions went beyond physical care. He explicitly attempted to medicalise drug addiction to shift blame from personal moral failures to biological chance:

> I feel like the psychosocial and counseling treatments are very important. The counselors I have a lot of respect for. But people get some message that there's a doctor involved in the treatment and it medicalizes it for them. It seems more legitimate than just going to groups or self-help. It relieves them. Like any illness, it's a socially acceptable [phenomenon]. Also I think that they like the explanations I try to give them. It's not like they're absolved from any responsibility for their choices. They're responsible for their choices, but their choices are also colored by their biology. Some of it's unfair. Everybody who is here probably started using drugs with someone else, a friend, or whomever. And lots of times that other person is not addicted now. They used drugs in high school and then they gave it up because they just did not have the protoplasm to become addicted. And this poor sap for some reason became addicted. It has been shown in research that one effective way to bring up the subject of substance abuse with people is to put it in a health context. You can tell them, look, not you're a bad person and this is illegal. It's more from the perspective of I'm your doctor. I care for your health. And for your health you should do this. I think that's been relatively convincingly shown that that seems to be less of a intimidating or the patients are more willing to accept. The message is the same but it's coming in a different format.

Here, the physician reframed addiction from illegal and bad behaviour to a health problem that required medical attention. This instance of medicalisation was consistent with the focus of the trial to find a pharmaceutical therapy for methamphetamine dependency.

Although every participant was required to undergo a physical examination and submit to medical monitoring, attendance at counselling was optional and inconsistent. Only a small number of participants finished the full counselling cycle, while most participants averaged two-three sessions. The staff explained the low attendance with participants' negative experience with peer-support group counselling:

We still have a lot of trouble with the counseling. People don't come. It hasn't seemed to be reflection of any new counselor. It's just that people don't come. Generally they tend to come to our studies because they're looking to get out of groups. And they're out of counseling because they've done...been there, done that, NA groups or whatever. And so they come here looking for the medication.

The counsellors did not consider the participants who failed to finish counselling failures but highlighted the small step of even going to counselling: 'I think of them as people who tried and then that try, they can build on whatever they got from that even if they came here one time. The fact that they made that step is a step towards success. So I don't think any of them are not successful. I just think that they're just along the wrong path right now.'

The counselling offered in the trial was behavioural-cognitive therapy grounded in social learning theories and principles of operant conditioning. In drug use treatment, this therapy emphasised functional analysis of drug use within a participant's life by looking at antecedents and consequences as well as skills training to recognise situations that may make people vulnerable to drug use, to avoid those high-risk situations, and cope when these situations are unavoidable (Carroll and Onken, 2005).

The participants who stuck with counselling saw benefits beyond their immediate drug problem. 'Like [the counsellor], she and I came up with things that would make me trigger. Okay, let's avoid those things. Okay, and then I found myself spending more time with my family because [the counsellor] added her input on what to do, how to do it, and try this, try that. That all – I don't know, it made me feel good. It made me feel real good.' They also hoped that the skills they acquired had longer-term utility than the medication. 'I'll be off of the medication eventually, you know. It's here today, gone tomorrow type thing, but the counselling's more effective to me. Maybe learning something, learning how to set and organise my life and keep it that way, you know, keep myself a routine.' Others simply saw the counsellor as a sympathetic listener to confide in.

The third treatment component of the trial was contingency management tied to clean urine samples. Except for the few participants in very dire financial straits, most respondents did not have strong opinions about the voucher system, thinking of it as a financial 'bonus.' The urine samples, however, offered a thrice-weekly statement of how participants were doing in the trial: 'I love it because, again, I am being held accountable. And right now I am not accountable to anyone.' Based on other drug addiction staff, the research staff thought that contingency management is motivational for some participants, even if they were unaware of it.

The final treatment option in the trial was the medication being tested. The prospect of a pharmaceutical that could take some of the edge off quitting methamphetamine was a great motivator for many participants. 'I figured like it would be kind of cool if they gave me a pill that made me stop wanting to use something to get high.' 'I'm hoping that this is a magic pill. I really am.'

Many of the participants hoped that the medication would be at least a partial substitute for methamphetamine. The physician in the study tried to warn against such interpretations: 'There's no magic bullet. You still have to really try hard. But the medication can help you, you know. It can help you do the counselling better, it can help you be more successful in the program. But it's not a substitute.' Other participants were afraid that the medicine would stimulate their cravings for methamphetamine: 'The pill, that worries me, you know, because I'm afraid if I get a little taste ...' Still others dismissed the medicine as an aid in their recovery: 'I could be taking gummy bears. I would have quit regardless.' The staff closely monitored participants for adverse effects, asking questions at weekly consultations. In addition, the staff lowered doses of the participants who complained about discomfort due to the medication. Participants who stopped taking the drug altogether were still allowed to finish the counselling and contingency management.

In sum, most of staff and participants' daily interactions centred around immediate treatment goals. The randomised clinical trial offered a set of four treatment components free of charge in confidentiality and with respectful staff. While not every participant appreciated all the components, most found something they liked. The trial as a form of treatment was particularly attractive in light of the few alternative treatment options available to people struggling with methamphetamine dependency. While this contrast makes the trial look good, it also reflects the weak treatment options for drug addiction in the US (Timmermans and McKay, 2009).

Outcomes: Research Toward Treatment

In light of the goal of finding a treatment for methamphetamine dependency, the bupropion study offered disappointing results. When the study was unblinded, the researchers found that bupropion only had benefited mild users. This was not even a hypothesised but a post-hoc finding, meaning that the researchers had not designed and sampled the study on severity of use. The researchers calculated five different aggregate measures of methamphetamine use but none of these showed statistically significant results. The low number of trial participants further weakened negative findings. Even more, some of the auxiliary hypotheses did not succeed. The only hypothesised positive result was that bupropion helped smoking cessation among the trial subjects: participants receiving bupropion smoked on average almost five fewer cigarettes per day compared to participants in the placebo condition. This was a minor positive finding for bupropion's efficacy.

Bupropion may increase seizure threshold and thus cause harm to patients with head injuries, making it unattractive in clinical settings. Thus the study director further weakened the utility of bupropion for mild users by imaging a clinician weighing the pros and cons of using the drug:

> To see the mild signal, everybody just kind of rolls their eyes, and thinks do
> I want to take the risk? Because for a clinician, they're thinking, I've got a
> bonehead in my clinic here. He's going to sit here doing some number of hits
> of methamphetamine, he probably has closed head injury. I'm going to be
> increasing seizure threshold, you know, for this much of a ... for a small amount
> of an effect size, you know, my question is, is it worth taking the risk?

In spite of the weak pharmacological effect, some participants in the trial
significantly cut down on methamphetamine or were able to quit the drug. Based on
the literature and similar studies, the physician involved in the study explained that
20–30% of trial participants were expected to improve based on the behavioural
treatments and placebo effects.

In addition, the tally of clean vs dirty urine samples masked others who cut
down on their drug use to a limited extent. As the physician in the study explained,
this effect had little currency outside the trial:

> We've had several people who did the whole study, had dirty urines every time,
> but cut down from injecting five times a day to, you know, twice a day, and
> some day zero. And that's actually a huge benefit for their health, and they're
> less likely to OD [over dose]. But for the medication studies, the only thing that
> matters is those clean urines. That's all anybody uses to judge the efficacy of
> medication. We collect all that stuff and we do analyze it. But when it comes
> right down to it, if you go to the meeting and put the slide up or you send the
> paper in, you know, people just do not care. The problem is that making those
> other intermediate outcomes better also hasn't always proven to be an indicator
> of them actually achieving. You'd think if you make depression better, they'd
> be more abstinent, right? But sometimes in several of the studies, people with
> improvement in their depression scores, they still didn't get clean anymore than
> people who didn't have the improvements in the person's scores. So from a
> quality of life perspective, you make them feel better, but the policy makers and
> the public, they want treatments to help people who want to stop.

Throughout the trial, staff and participants were pessimistic that anything would
stop methamphetamine addiction. Participants often had not only tried to quit
repeatedly on their own or through voluntary groups but they had experienced a
series of strong motivators to quit without result. Most participants had accumulated
financial losses and had to give up cars and homes. They had lost friends, partners,
spouses, and custody over children. They had lost jobs and promotions. They had
lost their teeth and other parts of their health. They also lost sexual drive and
self-respect. Some had been arrested and all knew that arrest for possession or
being under the influence of illegal substances was always a possibility. Most
of them wanted to quit but when asked how realistic it was that they would be
drug free at the end of the trial, they hesitated. A participant in the trial described
methamphetamine powerfully 'I call it "devil powder" because it slowly sinks the

hook in your ass and hooks you up.' In addition, participants were often familiar with other users who had tried to quit in vain.

Staff who had seen many people come and go were similarly pessimistic about the ability to treat methamphetamine addiction. 'I have a hard time believing that there's such a thing as methamphetamine recovery. The only way methamphetamine recovery would work is purely based on motivation. If you have a family at stake, that's pretty much your only hope of getting something out of programs, counselling, medications, placebos, whatever. That gives a little bit of a push, but the only way meth recovery is ... and I've seen it here as people that are on the verge of literally losing everything and it's the kids telling them, "Get treatment." That's the only way to go.' Staff members were unable to predict who would improve but sometimes unexpected 'miracles' seemed to occur. There was always hope but the staff did not have many illusions about its power to provide treatment. As the case manager put it, at best, she was a 'guide.'

In rare instances, staff took credit for the improvement of one of the participants. A counsellor felt that she had been influential in turning a young woman's life around:

> She was 26 and had been using for five years. The boyfriend was older and he was in jail. She didn't have a relationship with her dad. And part of the reason she was probably with these older people was her dad. And I just casually started talking to her about it and I said, 'Why don't you call him?' You love your step mom. Just hang out with your dad. And she started building a relationship with her dad. She started seeing her dad differently. Well, she started seeing herself differently. She started seeing herself as valuable. She enrolled in college. She's in the dorms. She got financial aid. She's still doing good. She ditched the boyfriend and told him he couldn't come back to see her. She built a strong relationship with her mom. She sees her dad every weekend. She's all right. I mean, she's going to make it, you know.

More often, however, the staff saw small behavioural changes, such as people 'coming out of their shell,' changing personal hygiene, or improving one aspect of their life.

At the unblinding of the study, the trial manager deliberately framed the study as successful for the impact the staff had on individual lives. While acknowledging that bupropion was a failed treatment, she drew attention to some of the successes on placebo.

> Of course, we know that the counseling does so much, and the contingency management does so much, and all of the rest of it, because it's been shown in previous studies, but the people who complied with the counseling did well. Whether it's the counseling or whether the fact that they were people who were invested in getting well is hard to tell, but either way, I mean, it does show that

at least the effect that it's important for them to come ... There were some really, really heavy users that got clean off the placebo ... That's huge.

The trial manager's intervention is to turn the placebo into a therapeutic study effect and thus attribute the successes on placebo to the staff's work. The end result of the study was thus that the drug had not fulfilled its promise, the majority of participants had not quit methamphetamine, but the trial had still produced some successes that could have been expected from contingency management and counselling. The trial confirmed previous knowledge about the power of psycho-behavioural treatments and indicated the limits of bupropion as an abstinence medicine. Finally, the trial confirmed that methamphetamine remained a powerful foe and that better treatments were needed.

Conclusion

Social scientists and journalists have scrutinised the clinical trial industry for its epistemic shortcomings and vulnerabilities. While social scientists include disclaimers that for some people pharmaceuticals may be helpful (Busfield, 2006: 299), it has become sociologically intuitive to critique this industry in a neo-liberal globalising world. Clinical trials have become epistemic instruments to establish safety and efficacy of potential blockbuster drugs but the social science literature contains many shocking stories of profit maximising at the expense of science (Healy, 2004; Fisher, 2009; Petryna, 2009).

While the risk that vulnerable populations will be exploited, demands oversight, Renée Fox drew attention to the routine intermingling of research and treatment in all aspects of medicine. Her analysis of the scientific team focused on ways of coping with problems stemming from the dual role of researcher and clinician. Physicians in the metabolic group faced methodological, scientific, and clinical uncertainties due to their exposure to the edges of medical knowledge. Interestingly, in subsequent research on medical education, Fox found a similar sense of uncertainty and the need for coping mechanisms among medical students, including the widespread existence of trial and error medical practice (Fox, 1957, 1980, 2000). More recently, David Armstrong (2006) observed that primary care physicians conduct mini clinical trials of their own patients to see how they respond to new medications, influencing the likelihood that they will prescribe these medicines for other patients. Even more, an experimental attitude runs through the debates about medicine as a science or an art (Berg, 1997) and evidence-based medicine (Timmermans and Berg, 2003). Here experimental discretion appears part of the professional prerogative of clinical autonomy, which, in the case of pharmaceutical prescribing, is the privilege to prescribe off-label. In the US, the FDA does not regulate physicians and it has been estimated that up to one-fifth of drugs are prescribed off-label (Radley, Finkelstein, and Stafford, 2006).

Much experimenting on patients is thus inherent to medical education and routine medical care but remains unrecognised.

In clinical trials, federal agencies explicitly regulate the link between treatment and research, which may result in a comparatively high-quality therapeutic set-up, as in this case. In the methamphetamine study this was evident in an interdisciplinary staff using state of the art treatment modules closely monitoring participants and invested in finishing the treatment-research cycle. The research infrastructure that allows for immediate follow-up of data points also produces a distinct form of care in which the clinical staff continuously reaches out to participants. Research and treatment converge on the shared goal of the participant doing as well as possible and continuing the full course of required services. These treatment characteristics are not incidental but deliberately implemented because treatment takes place in a research setting overseen by regulatory agencies who demand therapeutic benefits beyond the tested pharmaceutical. In the opinion of the researchers in the RCT studied here, the current set-up is more conducive to giving participants a high quality treatment experience than to maximise the likelihood that the research will produce positive results. Of course, it is important to keep in mind that the trial is superior to alternative treatments for drug dependency because these alternatives are not well developed. In an environment with high quality and easily accessible treatment opportunities, clinical trials would lose much of their attraction as therapeutic havens.

Chapter 2

Bridging the Ontological Divide: Different Social Worlds in the Conduct of a Pilot Study

Ben Heaven

The randomised controlled trial (RCT) is a collective enterprise requiring co-operation and a measure of mutual understanding amongst its contributors. However the priorities and expectations of those involved – from participant to trialist – may differ in important ways. To date a small body of qualitative work has explored the complex meanings expressed by participants regarding their involvement in trials, yet comparatively little research has extended this investigation to include the clinical and research teams involved. This chapter offers a rare insight into the work of a trial team as they negotiate research activities with busy practice nurses.

Drawing on a social worlds perspective (Strauss 1993), the insights of Friedson, (1988) and Traynor (2009) regarding the enactment of medical professions and Berg's (1997) writings on the construction and use of clinical protocols, I describe two social worlds engaged in the shared activity of a pilot study within an RCT. The worlds are defined here as: *RCT researchers*, represented in the activities of the pilot study by a small group of researchers – labelled 'the working group' – and a second world of *primary care practitioners*, represented by nurses recruited to the RCT. Although the pilot was intended as a collaborative enterprise, the reported priorities, meaning and actions of the members of these worlds varied considerably.

Context: The Research Environment

The 'diet-lifestyle trial' was a Health Technology Assessment (HTA) funded RCT comparing two different lifestyle interventions with medication, for the treatment of a common, chronic condition. The lifestyle interventions consisted of training packages for practice nurses, with the objective that the nurses use 'taught' skills and supplementary materials in consultations with participating patients. The lifestyle interventions differed: the first was a standardised advice package, and the second a personalised intervention based on the deployment of behaviour change counselling (BCC). The aim of the latter approach was to motivate the participant to change their lifestyle through encouragement and counselling, rather than via direct instruction. It was understood that changes in lifestyle behaviours might result in improved physical health, as recorded by each participant in a daily diary.

The purpose of the pilot study was twofold: (i) to develop and test the training materials in Behaviour Change Counselling (BCC); and secondly (ii) to measure the 'success' of the training via the degree to which relevant skills and materials were used post-training. One member of the working group – a dietitian – was given the task of developing and delivering BCC training in two clinic sites. Both practices recruited to the pilot study were known to be regularly 'research active', and few difficulties were expected in conducting the research at these sites. However once the dietitian began to implement the training programme, she encountered unexpected resistance and – at times – hostility from some of the nurses. In this chapter I attempt to explain the reasons for these difficulties. Centrally, I describe the *hidden work* of trialists in interaction with nurses. My aim is to illustrate the socially mediated and emotional nature of – what is routinely represented as – a dispassionate science.

The Pilot Study: A Promising Start

We might consider that practical problems of implementation are likely if the research question or the interventions themselves are of little relevance to their target population. However this was not necessarily true of the work described here. The research question itself was identified by the Health Technology Assessment (HTA) research programme as an area of importance for health research. In successfully bidding for funding, the research team produced a protocol that was carefully composed and researched. In addition, the topic area and the proposed intervention were both met with some interest in research and clinical communities. Investment in the trial therefore seemed to have been well placed. As the dietitian explained:

> I was an invited speaker at [a conference] ... my subject was [that of the trial] and I had a room full of 400 people who wanted to know about [the topic] and who were interested in what there was to be said ... and people [were] asking for the slides and ... asking questions and ... emailing questions so it's, you know, it's an area which causes people lots of problems, it causes practitioners problems because they don't know what to do with the people [with the condition] (Interview, Dietitian, 22.04.05).

As a member of the trial team one of the dietician's tasks was to train practice staff in the BCC intervention. A great deal of time was dedicated to the development of a training package for nursing staff based on BCC. Activities within the training sessions consisted of a general knowledge quiz centred on the chronic condition, its treatment and preventative behaviours. Information on treatment expenditure was also provided. The nurses were given specific instruction in BCC techniques reinforced by a DVD presentation. Finally they were given the opportunity to ask questions and give feedback. These sessions were designed to fit within the working practices of the clinical team. Across several meetings the working group discussed in detail approaches that would ensure the training avoided an authoritarian tone. Therefore, at the opening of the pilot study, the working group were poised for a positive interaction with practice staff.

Unexpected Difficulties

The working group encountered pronounced difficulties early in the pilot study. In the first recruiting practice the relationship between the dietitian and the nurses deteriorated to the point that delivering training became uncomfortable:

> It really shocked me, I got a *real shock* by the pilot ... because it had been fine and then suddenly when we were in that room [at a clinic site] and it was just so *overwhelmingly negative* and it was really, trying to stop myself from drowning for all 45 minutes and then we were basically chucked out of the room and I just didn't know what had happened all of a sudden, just a *breakdown in the relationship*, I mean why? So, because up until that point I thought that everything was alright but after that point I never wanted to go back in again, it took me a little while to get kind of get back down to normal and it took *a lot of persuading* to make me go back in (Interview, Dietitian, 22.04.05, my emphasis).

In this instance the dietitian made a very clear statement about the unexpected nature of the difficulties encountered in the pilot study. She explained that she 'got a *real shock*' by the hostility and '*overwhelming ... negative[ity]*' she encountered. Interestingly the dietitian describes the '*breakdown [of a] relationship*', suggesting that she had perceived an initial state of cooperation between the nurses and working group. However she also described being perplexed about the cause of the problem in this case. Finally the dietitian made an important allusion to the 'back stage' activities of the working group, when she noted that it took '*a lot of persuading*' for her to return to the practice (Goffman 1959). This left the dietitian with a problem: how to implement the training package whilst simultaneously managing relationships with the nurses. Success here could not be guaranteed by adhering to a protocol. Consequently the dietitian described feeling '*shock[ed]*' and '*overwhelm[ed]*' by rapidly becoming a key actor in the socially-mediated negotiations between social worlds.

A third and final problem for the pilot study emerged when feedback from the nurses and five participating patients suggested that none of the BCC techniques had been used post-training. In this regard the training for practice-based nursing staff had 'failed'. At the conclusion of the pilot study the working group reported that they had learnt a great deal from the difficulties of the pilot, and that consequently they had adapted their approach for the main trial. However a pertinent question remained: how was it that such difficulties were initially encountered, particularly considering the clinical and research interest, the involvement of qualified and experienced experts and detailed – and thoughtful – preparation?

Perspective of the Researchers: Negotiating Trial Interventions with an 'Unreliable' Audience

As representatives of the trial team, the working group held a shared understanding regarding the logic of the piloted intervention. This vision held them together as a collective. Essentially it was believed that the work of practice-based nurses could be enhanced through the use of BCC techniques, that deployment of such techniques might lead to a motivated patient – and thus to behaviour change – and that behaviour change could ultimately lead to improved health outcomes. The members of the working group were sceptical however that the link between nurse training and improved patient health would be free of contextually-bound interference. Indeed this concern developed throughout the interactions of the working group, holding them together as a collective, and eventually leading to their ideological departure from the larger trial team. Specifically the working group prioritised the issue of *fidelity*: the nurses' adherence to protocol. Consequently the working group expected some difficulties in translating their interests to the work practices of the nurses. At the conclusion of the pilot study I spoke with a member of the working group, a health psychologist, regarding her expectations for the intervention in the main trial. She noted, albeit with hindsight, that:

> … what we are hoping is that you know we are going to get lucky, the practitioners will change [by following protocol], the patients will change and the changes that they have made will make a difference to their [health complaint] so it's quite a mountain to climb I think' (Interview, Health Psychologist, 24.08.05, my insertion).

It is important to consider that the working group were enthused by the notion of developing both BCC-based interventions within the RCT, and a functional training package with possible broader application to primary care. Whilst each goal was subject to a different set of constraints, both were marked by tensions. The first issue was a desire to structure the nurses' behaviour within the RCT, whilst promoting the 'spirit of motivational interviewing' (p 20, subgroup: 1) which relied in part on tacit knowledge and contextually inspired, rather than rigid conduct. The second tension for the working group was the desire to promote BCC techniques as something new and exciting for the nurses, whilst acknowledging that differences in approach, whilst theoretically significant, were subtle. On a conceptual level this required both a problematisation of current practice – in order to justify the *need* for intervention – and a sympathetic understanding of the constraints that shaped it.

Within the research team, it fell to a dietitian to design and implement the training package in the field, with support from senior group-members.[1] However despite the experimental context of the pilot study, the dietitian was under some pressure for the training to be a success: both her clinical and research expertise were at stake. It is perhaps not surprising given this level of personal and professional investment, that the dietitian expressed quite strong views regarding the intervention. Indeed she displayed considerable frustration when the schema was challenged:

> If [the nurses were already communicating] effectively then there wouldn't be
> the health problems that there are (Subgroup 2: Dietitian, 03.02.04).

Whilst this statement appears cursory, it reflects closely the unified vision of the group. Moreover it is not a surprising perspective. Much of the literature regarding participation in RCTs is based on the same understanding: specifically difficulties in recruitment are often reported as having stemmed from the 'communication skills' of recruited clinicians (Wager, Tooley et al. 1995; Grant, Cissna et al. 2000). The majority of research in this area suggests re-skilling and re-educating clinicians so that their working practices are integrated more thoroughly with the precepts of the trial protocol. There is a certain irony then that whilst clinicians spend their professional lives communicating with patients, trial teams are comparatively inexperienced in these tasks. What appears to be a priority is meaningful communication between trialist and clinician, rather than clinician and participant.

The manner in which the training package was delivered may have affected the nurses' perceptions of the pilot study. Field notes from observation of the training session indicate that some problems had already developed between the working group and the nurses at an early stage in the study:

> This was the dietitian's second training session with this group of nurses [at site
> 1] … It was clear that the dietitian considered the [nurses'] choice of room on
> this occasion a comment on the training package: namely that [they] had chosen
> the small room as a form of resistance. In addition the dietitian informed me that
> two previous attempts at training had been unsuccessful. On one occasion she
> had been 'stood up' by the nurses once she arrived, and on a second occasion the
> nurses cancelled the meeting at very short notice.

---

1   The nature of the professional support in this context was both disciplinary based (through the guidance of senior dietitians) and clinical.

... [during the presentation] I noticed that the dietitian drew on her previous
clinical experience in an attempt to appeal to her audience ... [she discussed] how
the tool would have been useful in given scenarios. These were often prefaced
with: '*as a clinician* I found [x]' ... Nevertheless, my overall impression of
the training session was that almost all the nurses appeared to be bored ... or
sceptical of the BCC tool set. In addition I felt slightly uncomfortable as the
training package – rather than the dietitian's approach *per se* – felt somewhat
condescending. (Field notes I: observation of training session at site 1; 08.04
(day not recorded)).

There are a number of issues raised in the field notes that point to tensions between
the working group – or the dietitian specifically – and the nurses. In the first
instance the history of the relationship, as recounted by the dietitian, suggests
some resistance by the nurses to the training package.[2] Centrally, the account
indicates the dietitian's perception of growing tension across *several* encounters.
The account partially contradicts a previous assertion by the dietitian – cited above
– that there had been a sudden breakdown in the relationship.

In the second paragraph of the field notes I noted that the dietitian attempted
to present a clinical identity for herself and thereby, potentially, gain the support
of the nurses. Although it is not possible to ascertain if the dietitian's attempt
was successful in this instance, her actions reveal the presence of several social
worlds engaged in the pilot study: specifically that of the RCT researcher and the
sub-worlds of nursing and dietetics. As two potentially marginalised sub-worlds
within medicine, the nurses may have viewed the dietitian's attempt to gain kudos
as a 'fellow clinician' a futile or even inflammatory endeavour (Pope and Dowrick
2009, personal communication).

It would be misleading to suggest that the working group's initial view of
the nursing teams, as articulated in meetings, was particularly negative or
dismissive. Whilst the group clearly wished to meet their own needs in making
training attractive for the purposes of recruitment, their consideration of what they
perceived to be the needs and values of practice-based nurses was marked. They
saw the training as a novel package that would interest nurses and encourage them
to develop more sophisticated skill sets. However there was also a generally held
view throughout the working group that nurses in primary care could be resistant
to change and that they could take short cuts to the detriment of the investigative
process. A member of the working group recounted an experience in a previous
research project as an example:

---

2   One possible interpretation the events described by the dietitian is that they reflect
the realities of daily life in a busy practice: specifically that the nurses do not have time to
prepare a meeting room, and sometimes have to change previously made appointments.
However the dietitian did not interpret the nurses' actions in this way.

... [we] discussed some of the barriers within primary care settings, such as a common misunderstanding of research practices. One example given by the supervising dietitian was when a nurse asked if she could photocopy a completed questionnaire in place of administering a repeated measure, as the 'answers would just be the same'. The supervising dietitian explained that these misunderstandings can lead to clinicians viewing certain research practices as 'a waste of time', and as 'navel gazing' by academics, with the implication that researchers in turn view the involvement of some clinicians with unease and a measure of frustration (Field notes volume II: 31/10/05, RE: supervising dietitian interview).

The example above provides a classic example of an 'atrocity story': an attempt to position the teller of the story – in this case the senior dietitian – in a favourable light (Baruch 1981).[3] Atrocity stories are therefore useful rhetorical devices that perform some work in justifying courses of action.

... [T] he significance of ... atrocity stories lies in the way they establish the rationality of [the teller's] actions and also their ... reasonable and moral character. This is accomplished by appeals to standards of the everyday world which [the story teller] assume[s] are shared by the interviewer [or listener] (Baruch 1981: 276).

In the example of the senior dietitian's story, the working group were positioned as justified in doubting both the nurses' understanding of the 'science of the trial', and their likely fidelity to the interventions. Thus whilst the working group largely maintained a public 'front stage' concern with meeting the professional needs of practice-based nurses through the trial's interventions, at times a less positive view of nurses was articulated.

The problem of the pilot – to a greater or lesser degree – was perceived by the working group as resting with the nursing teams. From the perspective of the dietitian in particular, the key tension was that the nursing staff considered themselves *au fait* with the BCC approach. Of the two clinic sites used in the pilot it was the first which generated the most tension, culminating in an open argument in the waiting room. The degree of conflict completely confounded the dietitian who felt that she had done everything possible to make the intervention attractive. She explained:

... the barrier was that I suppose, ... [nurse 2] who I dealt with was just for some reason not that bothered or felt like she knew it all already and I don't think that when I did that presentation ... I could have put it more like a group

---

3   The concept of the 'atrocity story' and its application to this particular field note were drawn to my attention by a friend and colleague who kindly agreed to comment on a draft of this work (Rapley 2008, personal communication).

learning, I don't think I stood there as the expert, so there was just a bit of a, they obviously had a bit of a problem learning something which is just a reflection on her personality whereas other people in the group seemed to relate to it and not take it as 'this is what I am telling you to do' (Interview, Dietitian, 22.04.05).

However, far from being an isolated problem with a particular individual, the dietitian went on to find similar issues in the second site:

There didn't appear to be barriers [at the second site] because people turned up and re-arranged the next session there and then when I was in the meeting, but then I could sense from a few people that they thought it was full of, I was not kind of telling them anything, I wasn't giving them rocket science, erm, so again, but that's just the nature of the study you know it isn't rocket science (Interview, Dietitian, 22.04.05).

It is important to note the acknowledgement in the last section of the quote. There is some consideration of the subtlety between standard practice and the BCC approach, and how this might be perceived by the nurses as offering 'nothing new'. In this case, the value of the training is openly acknowledged as being less than 'rocket science'. In this brief moment, the dietitian almost takes the perspective of the nurses, potentially opening the way for improved interaction. However, emphasis remains on changing the nurses' consultation behaviour: that is BCC might not appear to be new, but that is not to say that it does not work. Interestingly, whilst there was some display of reflexivity within the working group at various moments, – usually in one-to-one interactions with the ethnographer – this did not lead to *action* in stopping the pilot, or discussing the weaknesses and feasibility of the interventions publicly. Toward the end of the pilot study the dietitian received critique from an external specialist, with expertise in BCC. The expert was – according to the dietitian – quite critical of her approach, leading her to express some anger. In particular the dietitian reported that having put work into her own training and attending courses, she had competence in the techniques. The rather ironic state of affairs – mirroring the experience of the nurses – was discussed 'off tape' and outside the working group meetings.

Perspective of the Nurses: Negotiating 'Poorly Conceived' Trial Interventions with RCT Researchers

My contact with the nurses recruited to the pilot study was relatively brief in comparison with time spent amongst the working group. Initially I accompanied the dietitian to her second training session in one site, and exchanged phone and e-mail correspondence with a senior nurse at the same practice. Later I interviewed nurses from both practice sites.

The nurses described their reaction to the training sessions in different ways but all agreed that the decision to participate had not been theirs to make. The choice of participation was ascribed to either one of the practice GPs or alternatively, a practice manager. Consequently practice hierarchy played a part in shaping the nurses' perception of the pilot study and training package. To further compound matters, the research team did not initially offer the nurses the possibility of working alongside them: the nurses were to be trained and monitored, and this power relationship was established however inadvertently, through the nurses' lack of decision making control. For some of the nursing staff this introduction to the trial was not unexpected or of great importance, whilst for others, particularly the more senior nursing staff, the lack of acknowledgement led to some resentment. Consequently the nurses expressed mixed feelings regarding involvement in the pilot, although all agreed that research involvement in general was important.

Two issues in particular appeared to encapsulate the nurses' concerns. The first was a conflict between the nurses' perception of their own clinical competence, and the challenge to this perceived expertise as represented in the working group's intervention. Whilst almost all the nurses expressed some willingness to learn new skills, they articulated a degree of uncertainty regarding the status of the training package. In particular several nurses commented that many of the BCC techniques matched their current skill set, and therefore questioned the value of the training. As one nurse explained:

> … [the dietitian] obviously had a good format, erm, and she went through it very very thoroughly, … and there was lots of time to ask questions, and, er, a lot of it was, maybe a bit teaching granny to suck eggs a bit because it was, er, … I think it was sort of based at the very basic level …I think some people might find it erm, to be a bit patronising, personally I didn't, erm, it was good, in one way it was quite nice to think oh I already do that or, you know that's okay (Interview, Nurse 1, Personalised arm, 08.09.04).

A district nurse based at the second practice vented some frustration:

> Erm the one thing I wasn't too keen on, was the role play that she did when the other chap came with her, I don't feel after 20 odd years of nursing I need to be told how to conduct an interview of any description, really. So that may be appropriate for less experienced people, maybe nurses who are coming into nursing or coming into these kind of jobs, but every single appointment I have I have to have interview skills for whatever the topic is and I know very well not to appear rushed and looking at my clock, not looking at my watch or the clock and that kind of thing (Interview, Nurse 4, Personalised arm, 11.10.04).

Some of the nurses described the working group as inflexible, attributing this to the protocol. For example one nurse described the BCC training as rather directive and simplistic. She commented:

> I don't suppose [the dietitian had] the luxury of quickly assessing her um, audience for want of a better word, and upping the pitch because *its a project* and I know with projects you tend to have to do, I mean I have done projects I have sort of done, been involved with quite a few diabetic projects, and often 'well you've got to teach it this way, because this is the project' you know, and, whereas if we were doing it, if I was doing it to a live audience anyway you know you can very quickly gauge from the feedback 'oh well this is too low I need to up it a level or I need to bring it down a level (Interview, Nurse 2, Personalised arm, 08.09.04).

The nurses viewed the protocol regarding BCC skills as prescriptive, and a poor fit with the tacit knowledge they routinely deployed in consultations. The idea of a free form, adaptive approach: – central to the BCC intervention – was quickly undermined as both parties attempted to interpret the interactional demands, and assumptions, of the other. Importantly in the third excerpt above, Nurse 2 is able to 'bridge the ontological divide', albeit briefly, when she demonstrates her understanding that '… you've got to teach it this way, because this is a project'. Unfortunately the 'pitch' of the intervention is described as being inappropriate for practice nurses: 'too low', and nurse 2 uses this to explain the disengagement of both herself and her colleagues.

A second, related set of concerns were grounded in differences between the domains of medical research and practice. Whilst the working group championed the concept of BCC as a novel, and potentially powerful tool in combating the chronic condition under study – condition 'X' – the nurses held a different assessment of the clinical problem based on their professional experiences. This assessment largely rejected patient motivation as instrumental to the improved health of the population under study. Hence several nurses expressed consternation at this emphasis within the training package:

> I think we kind of do [BCC] probably not quite so much as she was putting across. Certainly in other areas I do, because I do smoking cessation advice … but I think if somebody, if somebody comes to you with er [condition X] and you ask them how motivated are you to sort it out I think they would think you are a bit nuts, because they have come to you, 'will you help me?', 'well how motivated are you?' You know what I mean. … I feel just me personally, [I] wouldn't feel terribly comfortable saying that to a patient (Interview, Nurse 4, Personalised arm, 11.10.04).

Nurse 4 explains that asking patients with condition X about their motivation to change health behaviours would be '[un]comfortable' in comparison for example with smoking. She refused the trial team's vision: one in which practice-based nurses take on the work of managing condition X as a chronic illness. Indeed her account explicitly distances her from this role.

In summary, the personalised BCC approach was described by the nurses as a formal, explicit conceptualisation of some current practices for a range of complaints, but ultimately redundant in the setting specified by the trial team. Nurses described their routine work as a flexible adaptation to the realities of clinical practice and patient motivation. They cited patients who had either found satisfactory solutions to their symptoms through the use of readily available medications, or who lacked the capacity for significant behaviour change and required more direct intervention and guidance. In all cases the nurses identified their current practice as incorporating some of the BCC techniques and therefore did not reject the utility of the training outright. An underlying issue from their perspective was the working group's lack of insight regarding the clinical environment, the impression that their professional expertise was not recognised in the study design, and the working group's focus on protocol. In this sense the nurses saw the working group as staid and inflexible, ironically mirroring academics' beliefs about them.

The Participants: Evidence of a 'Failed' Intervention

Participation in the pilot study required that the nurses implement BCC techniques with a number of their patients. It was intended that the participants would then be interviewed by the ethnographer in order to ascertain the nature of the consultation, and ultimately whether the BCC techniques had been successfully deployed. Partly as a consequence of the tensions described earlier in the chapter, and partly due to time constraints, only five participants were visited by the nurses for the purposes of the pilot study. Subsequently only two agreed to be interviewed regarding these encounters. In both cases the quality of the collected qualitative data was poor, with the participants having very little to say about the consultation. Therefore the claims made in this chapter about the experiences of participants in the pilot study are limited.

In both interviews the participants described the consultations, and overall involvement in research, as mundane experiences. In this sense their reports echoed the sentiments of the nurses: the trial seemed to be offering 'nothing new'. However, it is important to recall that the nurses' reception of the training was not as envisioned by the working group. In their accounts the participants highlighted aspects of the consultations that confirmed some of the reservations of the working group. One participant (participant A, 10.11.04) described the interaction as: '... just like filling a form in', and '... [the nurse] asked the questions and I just answered them'. The working group interpreted the feedback from the participant interviews as confirmation that the nurses had resisted using a BCC approach. Further evidence was provided from materials used by the nurses and remaining participants in their consultations, and from interviews with the nurses themselves. Consequently the training intervention was regarded by the working group as a failure. 'Failure' in this context was a mistranslation of ideas and priorities from the world of RCT research to that of primary care practice. Nevertheless, from the nurses' perspective they had followed a simplistic and restrictive protocol and responded to an uninspiring 'intervention'. Therefore although the working group reached the conclusion that BCC had not been deployed, the nurses' indicated that they had met the obligations placed upon them.

Attempts at Creating Bridges

When delivering the BCC techniques the nurses were torn between competing expectations. On the one hand they were asked to perform as autonomous health professionals – including engagement in indeterminate work – yet simultaneously were required to act to a structured protocol. The BCC technique relied upon skills that appeared, *prima facie*, to be mundane. Consequently the dietitian's instructions for the nurses necessitated a pedantic explanation of an ideal social interaction in order to highlight the importance of particular phrases, gestures and suggestions that were key features of the BCC approach, and arguably of other aspects of nursing work. The nurses were therefore required to suspend some of their habitual practice, and shape their social and clinical interactions to the dietician's instructions.

The requirements of the intervention, to some extent, overrode the experience-based preferences of the nurses, and left them as 'instruments of the trial' (Rapley, May et al. 2006). However, as a profession, nurses are not unfamiliar with working to guidelines, protocols, and scripts for evidence based practices. Traynor (2009) notes that:

> Despite the danger that experienced nurses may find detailed instruction regarding certain mundane tasks insulting and absurd, many similar systems of cataloguing nursing activities, nursing diagnoses and nursing languages have been developed ... (ibid.: 504).

In the pilot study the nurses reported that working to a protocol for the purposes of research was not a key concern *per se*, as much of their routine work was structured according to various imposed constraints. Indeed Nurse 2, cited earlier in the chapter, made the point very clearly when she described familiarity in doing 'a project'. Centrally, the nurses questioned the working groups' problematisation of a chronic condition that was, in their experience, relatively 'unproblematic' in the context of routine primary care. The 'solutions' offered by the working group were perceived by the nurses to comprise aspects of their current training. Therefore two key issues were at stake: (i) a different understanding of the clinical 'reality' of the chronic condition and its management, and (ii) a clash between different social worlds – of research and clinical practice – compounded by tensions relating to the professional sub-worlds of nursing and clinical specialism's, namely dietetics.

Friedson (1988) offers an insightful summary of what was at stake for the nurses in these 'training' encounters:

> ... it is useful to think of a profession as an occupation which has assumed a dominant position in a division of labor, so that it gains control over the determination of the substance of its own work ... In fact, the profession claims to be the most reliable authority on the *nature of the reality* it deals with (ibid.: xv).

In this regard I have described a short trajectory of interaction between social worlds in which an ontological divide was revealed. However we may also consider the mobilisation of various professional bodies within the pilot which contributed to difficult – and emotional – social interactions in the pursuit of science, and attempts by both parties at bridging the 'divide'.

After initial reports of some unease amongst the nurses, members of the working group suggested a two-pronged approach to reposition the training package. The dietitian would ensure that the expertise of the nurses was formally acknowledged whilst asking for co-operation for the 'sake of research'. Potentially this opened the way for the nurses to take some ownership of the tools as collaborators in assessment, mirroring patterns – albeit on a much smaller and localised scale – reported by Traynor (2009) and Timmermans and Berg (2003) whereby professions gain an advantage through claiming formal tools as their own (Will, personal communication, April, 2010). The second aspect of the new approach was to ensure that BCC techniques were presented as a tentative approach to the clinical problem, rather than as a pre-determined solution: possibly creating space for the nurses to adapt techniques to localised concerns in a manner similar to that described by (Berg 1997). This approach would seem commensurate with the experimental context of a pragmatic RCT, and seemed appropriate to the working group. Moreover, the new strategy would achieve two objectives for the trial team: it might solve practical issues of implementation, and secondly would provide a formal and publishable account of what the working group had learnt from the pilot. However negotiations between the working group and nurses remained 'hidden' in formal reports. It is unclear from the data why this was the case, although we might speculate on a number of factors including: the seemingly 'mundane' nature of disagreements in collaborative research; the influence of passion in what is widely heralded as an objective and dispassionate science; and most pragmatically, the possibility that the trial would be undermined if the intervention was publically rejected by its intended users.

The responsibility for altering the presentation and ethos of the training package was delegated to the dietitian and she appeared somewhat reluctant to make these adjustments. In a later discussion the dietitian explained that as a clinician, rather than as a researcher, she felt uncomfortable asking the nurses to enact an intervention with uncertain efficacy. In particular, the proposed approach threatened to undermine concepts of efficiency and enhanced effectiveness which underpinned the 'selling points' of the research for busy clinicians. After interviewing some of the nurses it appeared that the dietitian's concerns were indeed attuned to some of their concerns. In my field notes created at the time of the discussion I wrote:

> [The dietitian] pointed out that she and her immediate supervisor had previously worked in the clinical environment, and therefore were well aware of the NHS 'culture' ... It seemed that in the conduct of the pilot the dietitian was caught at the intersection of two social worlds – that of the RCT researcher versus the primary care clinician – and that both worlds held competing interests and priorities. These concerns at the micro-level centred on what the intervention could achieve, and what it threatened, for each group (Field-notes volume II: 20.10.06, discussion with dietitian).

In this example it appeared that for the first time, the dietitian presented a potential bridge between social worlds. Here was, it appeared, the opportunity for an interesting dialogue between both parties. Throughout the pilot study there were other rare moments when both the dietitian and nurses moved independently into an intermediary space, considering the world view of 'the other'. One example of this is when a nurse reflected on the BCC skill set and how adoption of the skills might actually work, both logically and practically, to the benefit of patients. As she explained:

> Nurse 1: ... I tend to give advice rather than let patients come to their own decisions really, I tend, I would make an awful counsellor because I tend to jump in and try and sort out everything for them rather than allowing people to ... cope with the realisation that its down to them really ...
>
> Interviewer: right so ... in your experience of [clinical] practice do you think that that's really key ... it is their own realisation that people come to, to change their behaviour rather than giving advice?
>
> Nurse 1: yes, yeah because they will go off and take your advice, and they might do that for a while, but if it doesn't work, then they will come back ... where if you can change the pattern in the way that they are dealing with things then you know it's down to them, they can change their behaviour and lessen the contacts that we have! (Interview, Nurse 1, Personalised arm, 08.09.04).

In this instance we see the kind of response that might be perceived as justification for the BCC model. The benefits of a BCC approach are expressed succinctly. However the levels of complexity articulated by the nurses regarding differences between a model patient, and one actually engaged in routine consultation, have disappeared in this quote. The statement appears without qualifiers: the highly relevant descriptors that were raised throughout the nurse interviews about their own *practical activity*, and the 'reality' of clinical practice. Rather than justification for BCC then, we observe perhaps a concession, an attempt to see the positive in the values and beliefs of another.

Conclusion

Throughout the chapter I have discussed the activity of a trial team as they attempted to implement a pilot study involving nurses in two primary care practices. Specifically, working relationships between the nurses and the researchers responsible for the pilot – the working group – quickly became strained. Notably two key issues were central, both of which were deeply interrelated: the nurses and working group differed in their understanding of the value of the pilot study; and the nurses resisted what they perceived as challenges to their professional identity and role specification by external 'others'. Whilst the working group understood the pilot study to be a rational means by which to judge the training package – and ultimately the value of a change to clinical practice – the nurses interpreted the study through the 'reality' of their routine clinical work. Viewed from the nurses' perspective, participation in the pilot study gave them additional work for a condition that was a low priority and already well managed, and offered an intervention that, at best, was seen as elementary to professional nursing practice.

Conceptually the current chapter describes the collision of two social worlds, the practical activities that each world engaged in, the tensions that emerged from un-translated – or possibly untranslatable – concepts, and subsequent struggles to claim an essential 'truth' regarding the 'reality' of the pilot study. Both the working group and nurses were bound by the systems of logic embedded within their own social world. These logics were valid within their own contexts, namely those of research and clinical practice respectively. However in coming together in a shared enterprise these differences became problematic. At times individuals were able to reach across the ontological divide and understand, if only briefly, the perspective of 'the other'. Potentially these connections might have facilitated a *shared currency of understanding*, and the enactment of practical solutions. However, in the case of this pilot study few collaborative links were formed, and hence no real understanding across parties seemed to take place. It has not been possible to advance more detailed explanations of the divide that separated nurses and researchers here, not least because of an absence of data about the world of primary care practitioners. However it has been possible to illuminate the extent to which such differences were practically *enacted* – at times with emotion and passion – at the heart of what is typically seen as a dispassionate enterprise: the RCT. By exploring the occurrence of different social worlds and their inter-linkages we may gain a greater understanding of solutions to practical problems in the increasingly complex world of RCTs.

Chapter 3

From Dirty Data to Credible Scientific Evidence: Some Practices Used to Clean Data in Large Randomised Clinical Trials[1]

Claes-Fredrik Helgesson

Clean Data, Dirty Data and Data Cleaning

> There are cleaned data, but the cleaned set is not complete yet. The cleaning is under way. They have also to call sites and monitors. Stefan is, for instance, cleaning access databases. At data-management, excerpt from field-notes [055:001].

The excerpt is from a visit to a company specialised in data management services for large clinical trials. The company specialised in gathering, preparing and analysing data about patients participating in clinical trials and regularly performs these tasks for pharmaceutical companies. What piques my interest here is the term data cleaning, and the metaphors of dirty and clean data that comes with it. In a handbook of clinical trials dirty data is, for instance, defined as '… a collection of data that has not been cleaned, checked or edited, and may therefore contain errors and omissions. See Data cleaning.' (Earl-Slater, 2002).

Randomised clinical trials (RCTs) are often described as the gold standard for gaining scientific evidence about drug therapies. Given this strong position, it seems pertinent to take a closer look at the practices involved in solidifying their results. This chapter contributes to such an endeavour by focusing on how data is corrected and verified in large RCTs. Drawing on participant observation

1 The research for this project, 'Market and evidence', was supported by a research grant from The Bank of Sweden Tercentenary Foundation. Earlier versions has been presented at the workshop on evidence-based practice organised by Ingemar Bohlin and Morten Sager at the University of Gothenburg, 19–20 May 2008; at 4S/EASST, Rotterdam, 21–23 August 2008; and at EGOS, Amsterdam, 10–12 July 2008. This chapter has benefited from comments by a number of people who have read and commented different earlier versions. In addition to the participants at the P6 seminar at Technology and Social Change, Linköping University, I would in particular like to mention Ingemar Bohlin, Ben Heaven, Ericka Johnson, Tiago Moreira, Morten Sager, Catherine Will, and Steve Woolgar.

in different locales of large multi-centre clinical trials, the chapter describes a number of practices of data correction and verification. My investigation is guided by a few straightforward questions: How are corrections initiated and made? Who and what participates in making the corrections? And, finally, how is it recorded that a correction has been made? Behind these lies a broader inquiry into whether and how such cleaning practices might contribute to the credibility of the results produced by RCTs. Yet this broader inquiry should not be understood as aiming to unveil how allegedly unbiased results from RCTs may in fact be biased. Rather, I have a simpler and more profound aim: to contribute to our understanding of how the power of the RCT is constituted.

Locating Credibility: Formal Features of Large Pharmaceutical Trials

Trust, or rather the lack of trust, has been advanced as a key aspect in the emergence of the RCT after 1945 (Porter, 1995; Marks, 2000). Yet where Porter (1995) sees the emergence of RCT as a reaction to a lack of trust in pharmaceutical companies and physicians, providing a kind of impersonal authority for approving and assessing pharmaceuticals, Marks (2000) directs his interest to the inner organisation of RCTs. Marks argues that tools like the standardised protocol, untreated control groups, randomisation, blinding, and statistical testing all have been developed in response to a lack of trust in the different groups involved in performing trials such as patients, researchers, physicians and nurses. Porter and Marks agree however in pointing to the increasing credibility attached to RCT results – something which has intensified with the use of clinical guidelines, meta-analyses and health technology assessments.

The observations informing this chapter are made at so-called Phase 3 and 4 studies. These trials are typically large and long, in order to gather information such as the long term results of the use of the drug. There may therefore be more than a 1,000 participants, recruitment from several hospital clinics (sites in the RCT vernacular), which can be distributed across several countries. Increasingly these studies are coordinated by specialist companies, so-called CROs (Contract-Research Organisations), which have emerged during the last 15 to 20 years (Mirowski and Van Horn, 2005; Fisher, 2009). Other involved parties include researchers based at one or a few university hospitals, governmental agencies such as the medical products agency, an ethics committee and health care services organisations. Coordination is performed through guidelines and international agreements, rules, contracts and forms specific to the study, as well as rules associated with the pharmaceutical company (the sponsor).

As a rule, the staff at each clinical site identify potential patients and approach them to see if they are interested in participating in a trial. The clinic is also the place which the patient visits to receive the drug, give blood samples, and undergo investigations such as blood pressure measurement or ECG. Much of the routine work at a site is conducted by specially trained research nurses or biomedical technicians.

The data collected in a study are recorded on forms specially designed for the trial, Case Record Forms (CRFs). Everything recorded on a CRF is also to be recorded in the patient records or some other form that stays at the clinic. This allows for verifying what is recorded on the CRF against some other recording of the same data. According to Good Clinical Practice rules (GCP), the first place where something is recorded is the source data for that particular item of data and is to be kept at the clinic.

The records, files and other trial-related materials at a site are regularly examined by a so-called monitor, who comes from the CRO running the trial. They check that the data recorded on the CRFs are the same as the corresponding recordings in the patient records and other source data forms. He or she also checks other things such as that the documents are properly signed. The checks performed by the monitor also anticipate what would be examined by authorities such as the US FDA, if the trial and site were picked for an official audit.[2]

When the monitor discovers a deficiency or obscurity in the documentation she or he makes a note to the clinic staff asking them to resolve the issue. The monitor is strictly prohibited from altering the records themselves, even though they might have a very clear idea of what should be corrected and how. It is only when all such issues are resolved in a bundle of CRFs that they are gathered and sent to data management for further processing.

Taking an Interest in Cleaning and the Making of Credible Scientific Evidence

The current pre-eminence of RCT in medicine and health care makes it an important subject for investigation and discussion. One major topic in such discussions is how the results of RCTs may be inadequate or misleading (see, for example, Abraham, 1995; Abramson, 2004; Angell, 2004). In this literature, focus may be on ways in which the results might purposefully be biased through factors in the design of trials, for instance, through decisions about what patients to include and/ or the doses of different pharmaceuticals to be dispensed (see, e.g., Angell, 2004, 78–79). Such discussions address valid concerns about the RCT as a method for gaining knowledge and how it is practiced. Yet, research on bias accompanies a position that maintains the possibility of making a clear distinction between biased and unbiased RCTs. Such a position, then, would further maintain the possibility to perform RCTs where nothing unjustifiably and/or covertly shapes the data, and with results being the outcome of work strictly following rules, regulations and an unbiased protocol.

---

2 FDA also perform such audits at clinical trial sites outside the US.

A problem with taking bias as starting point is then that it frames any discussion about practice from a viewpoint that could be called a sociology of error (Bloor, 1976). According to this position, any idiosyncratic shaping of data should be understood as producing biased data and biased results. Here I want to do something different. I want to examine some normal and accepted practices related to the cleaning of data and see how they contribute to the solid credibility of the results produced by RCTs.

The focus on the practices of verifying and correcting data could be seen as looking at those activities that constitute what has been coined the regulatory objectivity of medicine (Cambrosio et al. 2006). Yet, my focus is not primarily on the regulatory side of knowledge production but how the actual practices of cleaning relate to, and deviate from, formal rules. This interest comes closer to Petra Jonvallen's study of two large clinical trials, where she observed and examined the large amount of local articulation work necessary in RCTs to be able to perform centrally prescribed activities (Jonvallen, 2005: 175–180).

Directing attention to what happens to data after initial capture and prior to the formal analysis is warranted not least since it appears to be under-examined in scientific research more broadly (Leahey, 2008; Sana and Weinreb, 2008). When this kind of activity has been discussed within science and technology studies, it appears often in relation to observations of researchers deliberately excluding certain data points with a purpose to alter the interpretation of data (see, for instance, Holton, 1978; Collins and Pinch, 1993).

Data from a Social Scientist

The data for this chapter mainly comes participant observation at different places where activities related to clinical trials have been performed. During my fieldwork I visited clinics and participated in patient visits. I further regularly visited an office of a CRO-company during one period, helping the staff with various tasks. I also took a two-day course for nursing staff on how to work with clinical trials. In all, my field-notes span more than 60 observations, where one observation is from a few hours up to a full day at a given site.

The observations are from a small number of drug trials within the field of cardiovascular disease. All sites visited are in different parts of Sweden. Nothing indicates that these trials were particularly well or badly run when compared to other trials sponsored by pharmaceutical companies. Informants sometimes remarked how sponsored trials differ from research funded trials in that they are larger, involve more rules and are more vigorously monitored. I was several times explicitly informed how a certain practice deviated from how it ought to be done, but that these deviations were the norm rather than the exception. It therefore seems plausible that what I observed represents mundane practice in a few properly conducted large RCTs.

Patients' approval was always secured prior to sitting in on their meeting with the physician and/or nurse. At the clinics I have also signed a promise of secrecy as regards the patients I met and the patient records I saw. I have also promised all who have agreed to my presence that the trials observed should not be identifiable in my reports, which puts some limits to what I can report. I have further chosen to render those involved in the trials anonymous. In this, I use the same convention for making up pseudonyms as Jonvallen, in which physicians are given names starting with a D (doctor), nurses are given names beginning with an N (nurse), and so on (Jonvallen, 2005: 64–65). The names chosen also reflect the gender of the person behind the pseudonym.

Capture and Correction: The Handling of Data at the Clinic

Source Data, Post-it Notes and Practised Principles of Disappearance

As noted above, according to GCP rules, the first place where something is recorded is the source data for that particular item of data. According to these rules, the source data is to be kept at the site making it possible to verify the corresponding CRF page against this primary recording. Each study has a list of what should be source data for different pieces of information. Sometimes the GCP definition of source data can come in conflict with the practices of capture and the study-specific rules. Nina told me that a nurse's hand could become source data according to GCP, if, for instance, a patient's weight was jotted down there first. Other, less unwieldy, objects can also become source data in opposition to what is stipulated for a given trial:

> Nina [nurse] points out that [scribbles on] a yellow Post-it note can become source data. She continues affirming that one have to keep such things out of sight of the monitor, saying instead [to the monitor] that the information was first recorded in the computer [i.e., the appropriate place for this data] while keeping a straight face. On site, excerpt from field-notes [007:001].

What Nina suggests, then, is that improper source data such as a scribble on a Post-it note is best made to disappear before the monitor arrives for the recurrent examination of the records. Instead a prescribed repository, such as a computer record or a designated form, are made to play its designated role as source data for that particular item of information.

The same stance was also manifested by a seasoned monitor while discussing with a nurse who was in the early days of her first trial. When going through a binder with patient data, the monitor explicitly made a distinction between what the GCP-rules prescribed and what would be workable:

> Monica [monitor] reads a printed page from the patient record that Natalie
> [nurse] has printed. She says [to Natalie]: 'you have all three blood pressures
> here' [in the record]. She stresses that this is good. 'Yet, if you were to first
> scribble them on a little piece of paper, that would be source data according to all
> GCP-rules, but that is not the way to do things.' [To keep these pieces of paper
> in the binder.] On site, excerpt from field-notes [023:001].

The monitor here in effect initiated the nurse in an apparent common deviation
from the GCP-rules. In practice, source data is tidy recordings of data that can
be made to appear as the first place where the data has been recorded. Possible
less tidy first recordings of data, such as scribbles on Post-it notes, are to be
cleaned away before the monitor arrives. A similar technique of applying Post-
it notes, which later disappeared, was also used by the same monitor when she
had questions or in some other way wanted the site staff to do something with
the records. Sometimes the issue in question was briefly noted on the Post-it note
itself, such as 'signature!' indicating that a signature was lacking.

> Monica [monitor] tells David [physician] that regarding the first patient [files]
> she checked it was noted hyperlipidemia in the patient record but not in the
> CRF. David checks in the binder. There are four small yellow Post-it notes in the
> binder at various places, each indicating a question from Monica. (On most of
> them she has made a note.)

> Natalie [nurse] then removes a Post-it note that Monica has put there [on a page
> in the binder]. // I say to Natalie that Monica went crazy when David earlier
> had removed such notes. Malena wants to see where she has pointed out issues.
> Natalie then becomes unsure if this should hold also now. She decides, finally, to
> leave the note there, but makes a scribble indicating that the issue is resolved.
> On site, excerpt from field-notes [037:001].

The last part of the excerpt above shows how Natalie was about to clean away
Post-it notes as a reflex action and how I intervened since I had heard how irritated
the monitor had been when the physician earlier had begun to remove precisely
these notes. Here the yellow notes in the binders represented a kind of order for
the monitor, whereas above the same kind of notes represented disorder in terms
of actual source data that the monitor to did not want to see.

   Yet, at some point even the monitor's Post-it notes must be cleaned up. Indeed,
their value comes precisely because they facilitate cleaning that leaves few traces.
Two days before the encounter with the Post-it notes used by the monitor I observed
the following:

> Monica shows me a form, a log, for where she as a monitor can note all issues
> she finds when examining the binders and forms at the site. She says that she
> does not use it since it is tiresome to use and that it is far simpler to use yellow

Post-it notes. David was, she continues, nevertheless stupid when he removed such notes on the pages where he had acted upon her questions. She says that she wants to keep them there so that she can verify that the issues have been resolved properly. She ends by stating that she will make a point [to David and Natalie] that they should let the Post-it notes stay put. On site, excerpt from field-notes [036:001].

By using Post-it notes instead of a log, Monica was able to find the pages where she had pointed out deficiencies or obscurities for the site staff to act on, and easily show them where these issues are located. This is important since the monitor is not allowed to make any correction him or herself no matter how simple. Using notes, she could communicate what needed to be done, while not doing it herself. Another feature of this practice is that the monitor can make the notes disappear when tidying up the binders after having verified that the issues are resolved. Then there is no log of once outstanding issues. The only trace of the cleaning are the scattered places where a correction is indicated by striking through the earlier data, entering the new data and adding a signature and date to indicate the change. (It is not allowed to erase an old recording.) At one point these Post-it notes allow for communication between monitor and site staff. When their work is done, they are made to disappear making it impossible for the site staff, the monitor and indeed any external auditor to get an overview of once outstanding issues.

Practices for Finding Deficiencies and Making Corrections

What, then, allows for identifiying deficiencies in the data? A large variety of things can be found by the monitor as warranting a correction or clarification from site staff. It may be a piece of information recorded in one place, such as in the patient record, but not recorded in a CRF. It may be a signature on a form that is missing. It may also concern recorded information that the monitor suspects to be wrong. The same day in the field I noticed, for instance, the following discussion between the monitor and the nurse:

> Monica asks Natalie about a patient. It says in [the CRF] that he has taken 'simva' (simvastatin) the same day as the visit. They conclude that simva is usually taken in the evening and that the patient hence had not taken simva the same day prior to his visit. Monica puts a yellow Post-it note on the page [indicating for the site staff that they should change this]. On site, excerpt from field-notes [036:001].

The deficiency made out here was a question about whether a patient had taken a pharmaceutical prior to visiting the clinic for leaving blood samples etc as claimed. The pharmaceutical in question is regularly taken in the evening and this is also what is recommended for this drug. It would furthermore be inappropriate for the patient to have taken the pharmaceutical shortly before leaving blood samples.

Here the monitor and the nurse discuss the matter and agree that the original recorded information was probably incorrect. The outcome of their discussion is that the page in the patient binder receives a yellow Post-it note, requesting the physician to make a correction on the CRF.

The most commonly found deficiencies were of a simpler kind such as signatures missing or discrepancies in how the same data was recorded in two places. The latter kind concerns, for instance, times when a data point recorded in a CRF did not correspond to the same data point noted in the patient record. Such discrepancies are routinely searched for by the monitor and vigorously noted. This practice of verifying data points against one another is a major route for identifying deficiencies and asking the staff to make corrections that align the records. This work also prepares the records for verification in a possible external audit.

In the above I have discussed instances where deficiencies are identified by the monitor looking at the records and perhaps interacting with site staff. In these cases possible corrections involve only the site staff and the monitor. Moreover, if the monitor refrains from using a detailed log, there will be few traces beyond the changes made to the particular form. The story becomes more complicated when the suspicion of deficient data is raised at the offices of the CRO or data-management. Here the verification of the data on can include automated checks of different forms concerning the same patient against one another and checks for outlying values. When something suspicious is found, such as a value on a CRF that is outside set limits, a Data Clarification Form (DCF), is issued to the site asking them to confirm or correct the suspicious value. Further on in the trial referred to above, Monica told me how the sites were beginning to receive DCFs in response to receiving CRFs from the clinics:

> Monica [monitor] tells me that data-management ... now has begun to send out DCFs. They are sent by fax directly to the concerned site, but she gets a copy by mail as a PDF. She tells me that some concern tiny issues. The limits for asking about weight, height and blood-pressure were initially set very tight, which resulted in many questions. // She further tells me that there are also matters that both she and the nurse have missed. It can, for instance, be that they have failed to indicate on what arm the blood pressure has been taken. She provides an example of a site where they both [she and the nurse] have missed that for a number of people. She further adds that when she begins to receive DCFs, she takes note of what they concern in order to avoid further DCFs on the same issue in the future. On site, excerpt from field-notes [054:001].

The use of DCFs obviously makes the documentation of possible confirmations or corrections more overt than when corrections are made directly at the site. It is further worth noting the role of set limits for identifying the suspiciously deficient. At a few instances I even came across a practice where a site stressed that a value that could be taken as suspicious actually was correct with the aim of countering a future DCF on the matter. The remark Monica made about trying to adapt to avoid unnecessary DCFs tells a similar story. Indeed, it indicates how the DCFs can shape more local cleaning practices in general. Avoiding DCFs is not only a matter of avoiding a nuisance, as the number of DCFs a site receives is also used to assess the proficiency of the monitor responsible for the site.

Who does what at the site? On the distribution of tasks and powers to make corrections I have already touched upon crucial distributions in who can do what, such as the rule that monitors are prohibited to make corrections themselves. There are further distinctions about what CRF pages may be filled in and corrected by either nurses or physician-investigators. These distinctions are manifest, but not as absolute as the distinction between the monitor and the site staff. One example occurred during the session involving the monitor Monica and the new nurse Natalie. For one correction they concluded that it was such a minor one that Natalie could do it herself, although it was a CRF related to pharmaceuticals and in that sense the territory of the physician. In the case when the patient had taken simvastatin, however, they concluded that it was a correction the physician had to do himself and restricted themselves to asking him to make it.

At the sites, I frequently saw how the monitor could provide very firm guidance on how a certain CRF should be filled in or how a correction was to be made. A number of these have also been described above. On a rare occasion I saw the monitor go the tiny step further to actually enter something on the CRF herself. This was in a situation where the monitor was going through a number of difficult pages together with the physician-investigator at the closing of a site at the end of the trial. Instead of having to go back to the physician at a later time, she postponed the filling out of the form to when she had the necessary information:

> Malena [monitor] then says that she is uncertain whether it is to be marked as a Serious AE [Adverse Event] or not. She says to Dustin [physician]: 'If it is ok with you, I can tick off the right box after having talked with "safety" [a special department at the pharmaceutical company].' He says that it is ok, and signs the CRF-page with this bit of information yet to be filled in. Excerpt from field-notes [052:001, p. 6].

In this specific situation Malena had prepared what the physician was to fill in on several different forms, but had not been able to establish what was to be ticked on this specific form. She further remarked to me that preparing what to fill in was ordinary practice, but that the filling in herself was truly violating how things ought to be done. (When subsequently making the appropriate tick, she was careful to choose a pen that had the same ink colour as the pen the physician had used when signing the form.)

Further Cleaning the Data at the Data Management Office

Working Towards a Clean File to Break the Code

The data management function is where all the CRFs are entered into a database alongside other information about the patients (such as the possible endpoints as well as data from the lab tests of blood tests taken). An important part of the work here is to check and correct the data. In short to clean it. The cleaning is done through various means, and the issuing of DCFs from data-management has already been touched upon. Below, I will provide some further examples of cleaning done at such a place based on a visit to the data management services firm mentioned in the introduction.

A major part of the work of cleaning at this data management office consisted of comparing different records and trying to eliminate any deviations and inconsistencies found. One example I observed concerned the results from a laboratory. In this case the lab data was registered to a patient-ID (unique number for each patient in the trial) that did not correspond to the birth-date and patient initials noted on the same sheet. The investigation then tried to decipher the right patient for this data.

The corrections of the data are done on a blinded data-set, meaning that no one at the office could see what specific treatment an individual patient had been given. This practice of 'breaking the code' only when all data was clean was emphasised during my visit:

> Everything they do now is run on blinded data. The unblinded database is safeguarded. They are very careful in stressing that. They only connect to the unblinded database after they have declared *clean file*. Now there are reports on outstanding issues sent to monitors [and sites]. At data-management, excerpt from field-notes [055:001].

For the trial they were working on, they ran some 200 edit checks on the data from the CRFs entered into a database. These checks caught outlying data, which could then be checked against the original CRF or indeed the source data if the paper CRF also contained the outlier number. This is, thus, a means of making DCFs to send to the clinics for correcting or confirming the odd data point (cf. about receiving DCFs at site above).

Not all corrections warrant involvement of the clinics, however. Some parts of the cleaning concerned standardising and coding what the physicians had recorded in open-ended fields on CRFs. 'People cannot spell. There are at least 100 different spellings of headache...'[3] as one informant told me and continued to describe how they used software to set the same code to different spellings

---

3   At data-management, excerpt from field-notes [055:001].

of a word. They assessed that some 90% of the terms could be corrected using automated algorithms, where the rest warranted a more manual treatment.

Making Judgments When Correcting Data at the Data Management Office

In the previous examples, corrections were either automated or deferred to the clinics using DCFs. At the data management offices I also came across situations where more explicit judgments had to be made regarding the quality of data and what actions to take. One such incident concerned whether the issuing of a DCF was necessary or not. This case resulted from an ambiguous recording of the date for a set of blood samples, and the staff deliberated on whether it was necessary to investigate the issue further:

> Stefan [statistician] and Carina [manager from the pharmaceutical company sponsoring the study] are discussing a date for a patient visit where blood samples were taken. It says April (a given year), but it is unclear if it is 2 or 12 April. I hear Carina stating that she could take on the responsibility for setting April, but not for going further. They continue discussing of whether to set 2 or 12 April, almost like it was a negotiation. At data-management, excerpt from field-notes [055:001].

I do not know whether this ambiguously recorded date resulted in the issuing of a DCF or not. Irrespective of the outcome, it illustrates that issuing a DCF to assist in the correction of data can be at the centre of professional discussion and judgment.

Another instance where judgments were openly called for concerned the interpretation of ECGs. For this trial a procedure had been set up where all ECGs taken at the trial sites were examined and coded by two nurses. Their two individual assessments of each ECG were subsequently examined by a professor in medicine who determined the final coding of the ECG. These assessments were hence made quite removed from the various sites where the ECGs had been taken.

When I visited the data-management office I heard of an instance where the nurses and the professor had reached a conclusion about two ECGs that overrode what the staff at the site argued:

> Another case on Cecilia's [project co-ordinator] desk is one where both the coders have assessed that the ECG from 2000 and the one from 2005 have been taken on two different patients [despite them being identified as stemming from the same patient]. Professor Pettersson has also concluded that these two ECGs are from two different patients. The investigator [the physician at the clinic] has, however, affirmed that they indeed are from the same patient. Cecilia says that the more recent ECG has to be removed from the trial data. This makes the earlier ECG from this patient valueless. At data-management, excerpt from field-notes [055:001].

In this instance, then, the judgements made by the two nurses and the professor corrected the data by exclusion. Their judgments carried more weight than affirmations of those who had participated in taking the ECGs.

Reflecting on Dirt and Perfection

Several of my informants reflected on the sources of errors and how to make the corrections. Some such themes has already come across above, such as the emphasis on balancing the formal rules against a pragmatic stance as to what is workable. Perfection is another such theme that warrants special consideration. This theme includes the notion that perfection is impossible. At the same time, then, as the abundance of small deficiencies and obscurities are deemed undesirable, they are viewed as a natural part of the everyday practices of clinical trials:

> Malena [monitor] then says: 'There are many sources of errors in this, but that is the way it is in studies with people involved.' She expresses the necessity to be pragmatic several times during the day, and that it is impossible to do everything to perfection. At the same time she emphasises that this particular site has not been run in a good way. At site, excerpt from field-notes [052:001].

Another side of this theme on perfection is that apparent order is suspicious in itself. According to this reasoning, perfection was a sure sign of fraud. One story about a clinic where all data for the trial contained no obscurities or deficiencies was told at the course I took. I brought it up when managing the messy site with the monitor Malena:

> In relation to this [the many queries] I tell Monica [monitor] about the GCP course I took where they had said that nothing can be perfect (without queries). Monica tells me that when she took such a course they had told her about a perfect site. All bottles of pills, binders, etc. was perfect. Yet, the patient records were always somewhere else (the physician ambulated between two offices.) The data was invented. With monitor at site, excerpt from field-notes [052:001].

Another monitor, Martin, told me another story about a clinic where data had been fabricated and where they had been tasked with rerunning the analyses excluding the data from that particular clinic. He also relayed the same notion that perfection should raise suspicion. Data that is clean all by itself is indeed the dirtiest data of all. Data, on the other hand, that requires work to be corrected, confirmed and aligned, is on the other hand dirty in a proper and authentic way and can become cleaner through such work.

Distributed Cleaning and Concentrated Results

There are, as I have aimed to illustrate, many different practices within large clinical trials that in one way or another contribute to making data clean. Entries like 'headake' and 'heddache' on CRFs all become headache in the database thanks to practices involving algorithms for standardising data. Data on CRFs are verified against source data recorded in, for instance, patient records before being sent to data-management. If the records do not match, corrections are made to align the two.

I will in this concluding section first summarise my observations regarding how corrections are initiated and made, who participates in making them, and how the acts of correction are recorded. Second, I will relate these observations to the issue of how these practices of cleaning might resemble and differ from practices that can make data dirty. Thirdly, and finally, I venture into the broader question about how these cleaning practices might contribute to the credibility of the results of RCTs.

Initiating, Making and Accounting for Corrections

It is striking how many of the different correction practices observed were initiated by identifying peculiarities with references to standards and norms. An obvious example of this is the identification of strange spellings. Another example is how data outside set limits for things like height, blood pressures, and so on are found potentially faulty warranting an extra confirmation. Another, somewhat more intricate route for identifying peculiarities is the comparison of the data with rules and recommendations. The example where the nurse and the monitor concluded that the patient had not taken simvastatin in the morning before the visit is of this kind. Here general recommendations worked together with the inappropriateness of the drug having been taken before the visit.

Problems might also be identified by comparing records to see if some data recordings stand out as peculiar. The most frequently observed example of this was the verification of CRFs by comparing them with the source data, but there were others, such as the comparison of two ECGs performed by two designated nurses and a professor. There are, then, a number of ways in which data can appear peculiar warranting a further confirmation or indeed a correction or exclusion. At the same time, though, the routes used to find such peculiarities do not involve questions about what happened when the source data was captured. Indeed, revisiting the initial act of capture is rare even when a data point is found to need correction. Instead other referents are used both for identifying peculiarities and for informing what corrections to make.

One pertinent aspect of these observations is how close techniques for problematising data are to the routes for verifying them. In some parts they are indeed inseparable, such as when the monitor verifies CRFs by comparing them to the source data and pointing out to the staff where corrections are warranted.

When a verification fails due to an inconsistency, the correction habitually consists of making the two records the same. Values outside set limits are further given an extra check and data that appear odd in relation to established rules might also be edited.

The outcome of this work is therefore a more aligned and consistent set of data, and this becomes the definition of clean data. The cleaned data would further better stand the scrutiny of a potential external audit, which would have to rely on the same routes as those used to make the data clean. At the same time, though, the very presence of obscurities and deficiencies seem to provide a comfort to those involved that the data is authentic rather than fabricated.

There are many kinds of persons and devices involved in the work to identify peculiarities and make corrections. In the examples provided above standards, patient records, algorithms, orthography, recommendations, nurses, physicians, monitors, statisticians, and a professor have all played a part in cleaning data. Apart from the striking diversity of 'cleaners', however, it is worth reflecting further about the distribution of cleaning work between locales of a trial.

One such spatial aspect is the inclination to keep cleaning as local as possible. A nurse, having first captured some data on a Post-it note, is inclined (and indeed encouraged) to clean improper source data repositories away after having transferred the data to the correct form for source data. The monitors, in their turn, are inclined to find and weed out obscurities so that they do not turn up in the form of DCFs from data-management. Even at data-management, I observed an instance where staff were deliberating as to whether they could set a correct date themselves or whether it warranted a DCF and the involvement of the site staff. This propensity of keeping cleaning practices local makes the term invisible work truly appropriate in this context (cf. Star 1991). There, seem, moreover to be both gendered and hierarchical aspects to this propensity to 'disappear' this work.

Pointing out the local aspect of cleaning should not, however, be taken to mean that it is spatially isolated. Standards, norms and recommendations can readily be seen as enrolled in invisible local work of data cleaning. The propensity to keep it local does however show up in relation to transfers of requests for corrections, which takes us to the issue of recording such corrections. Efforts to avoid unnecessary DCFs are a prime example of the preference for correction to be kept local, as well as the use of Post-it notes, rather than a log, to mark out deficiencies. One feature of this 'disappearance' performed on the very acts of cleaning is important: the outcome of cleaning – the aligned and consistent data – does not fully bear the story of its own cleaning. Generally the marks of the acts of cleaning are kept more local than the cleaned outcome.

What might Distinguish Practices of Data Cleaning from Practices making the Data Dirty?

It should be clear from the above that cleaning means the data become further shaped and formatted by influences from outside the situation of initial capture.

This includes such matters as recommendations, professional and idiosyncratic judgments, as well as notions of what are to be expected values. Given these many varied elements involved in the cleaning, one could possibly argue that the cleaning itself might introduce rather than eliminate errors and omissions.

Yet, it is here that the power of the aligned and consistent outcome of the cleaning begins to become evident. The clean data consists of fewer distinguishable errors and other peculiarities. In the introduction I cited a handbook of clinical trials that defined dirty data as data that had not yet been cleaned, checked or edited. The importance of the invisibility of much cleaning work also now becomes more apparent. The cleaning clearly contributes to producing data with relatively few distinguishable errors, but leaves at the same time not that many visible marks of its own work.

Practices that make data dirty would hence be different from cleaning practices in two dimensions: they would produce more distinguishable errors and omissions and this work would be more fully recorded and accounted for. Yet, such practices would probably share with cleaning practices a reliance on such things as recommendations, professional and idiosyncratic judgments, as well as notions on what are to be expected values.

How might Cleaning Practices Contribute to the Credibility of the Results of RCTs?

RCTs are seen as methodological gold standard for gaining scientific evidence about drug therapies. Their results are generally considered extremely credible. This strength makes it pertinent to take a closer look at the practices involved in solidifying the results of RCTs, and in particular into whether and how cleaning practices might contribute to the power of the results produced by RCTs.

In the previous sections I have gradually built an argument that the important outcome of the cleaning practices is a more aligned and consistent set of data and that the work to achieve this is far more extensive and multifaceted than what is accounted for in formal accounts of trial methodology. I have, in addition, stressed how the need for such cleaning work in itself makes the data more credible in the eyes of those involved. Adding this together suggests that the cleaning practices contribute to the credibility of the results of RCTs in two distinctly different ways: to those involved, the apparent need to clean, certifies that the data is authentic. To others, the cleaned data certifies that the trial's data is the ordered product of work adhering to formal procedures. This later effect then, is in no small part due to the data bearing few visible marks of provisional cleaning. In the end then, the clean data appears as authentic and the ordered outcome of formal procedures, a powerful combination that contributes to the credibility of the RCT and its results.

PART II
Framing Collective Interpretation

In this section, two chapters address alternative forms of data work that emerge in the process of the interpretation and evaluation of trial data – its messy afterlife. Both address institutions and moments beyond the actual implementation of a trial protocol, but continue to reveal the importance of professional politics, and of efforts to account for the relationship between research and practice.

The focus for Will is the effort put into assessing the meaning of commercially funded pharmaceutical trials, as instantiated in the pages of professional journals from the US and UK. Here editors and clinicians acknowledge that the bare mechanism of the RCT is not sufficient to discipline the activities of industry. Though correctly carried out research produces certain knowledge, or perhaps better, reduces areas of uncertainty, trials can be used by pharmaceutical companies to engage in subtle forms of 'agenda setting' in terms of the direction of research, clinical practice and guidelines. The peer-reviewed journal appears to offer such agendas a powerful source of credibility, here accompanied by efforts to mitigate or modify them with reference to other forms of knowledge. For Moreira such efforts appear in the process of a cost-effectiveness appraisal carried out by the National Institute for Health and Clinical Excellence (NICE) in England and Wales, and a legal challenge to that appraisal from patient groups and industry.

In both cases, professionals and other collectives work to identify the gaps remaining on completion of robust experiments. Initially for Moreira this relates to cost utility: economists seek to provide models derived from trials to make judgements about the effective use of national resources. However as their conclusions work to limit the use of new drugs for Alzheimer's to particular patient groups, other information about the value of pharmaceutical treatment, and the difficulties of patients and their carers, are brought into the public eye. This does not prevent diverse groups accepting trials as authoritative sources. Indeed, clinical resistence to NICE's guidelines is ultimately justified with reference to narrow accounts of trial conclusions as a defence against the cost models. Similarly in the case described by Will editors accept the importance of trials and offer models of 'critical appraisal' of their methodological adequacy. However they also argue that understanding the meaning of trials requires additional knowledge, for example of physiology; of the complexities of practice; of real-life patient populations; of the place of chance in a single experiment; and of gaps in the evidence base because of trials that cannot and will not be done. Efforts to restrict the potential for journals to become the mouthpiece of industry therefore rest on articulating very diverse forms of knowledge in this particular 'public' space.

Chapter 4

Addressing the Commercial Context: The Collective Critique of Clinical Trials

Catherine Will

'If Richard says it, I'll listen.' A single sentence from an interview with a primary care physician says much about the status still enjoyed by some medical journal editors. In this case my respondent was talking about Richard Smith of the *British Medical Journal* (BMJ) but at the time he might equally have been referring to Richard Horton of *The Lancet*, another journal with an international readership. For the general public too, editors like Marcia Angell from the *New England Journal of Medicine*, have emerged as personalities in the past decade, putting a face to widespread anxieties about pharmaceutical industry funding of clinical research and its dissemination (Angell, 2004). Yet academics, both social and clinical scientists, remain pessimistic about the ability of professional journals to mitigate the effects of this commercial context.

Though the influence of Evidence Based Medicine (EBM) has helped ensure that trial results have become more important for public policy and clinical practice in the last twenty years, most of the funding for these trials still comes from the private sector, i.e. the pharmaceutical industry. This chapter explores efforts to educate ordinary clinicians about the ways in which such trials may be 'biased' but also work more subtly as forms of 'agenda-setting' for their sponsors. Its particular focus is the medical journal, and attempts to make this a site for collective appraisal of trial data. Can this professional critique provide an adequate defence against what social scientists have called 'corporate science'? What kinds of knowledge are marshalled in the attempt, and how are they given credibility?

In seeking to answer these questions, I draw on the concept of 'epistemic culture' developed by Knorr Cetina (1999), exploring the use within medicine of what she calls 'negative knowledge'. In her account, developed from ethnography with high energy physicists, this relates to the ways of thinking about 'the limits of knowing, of the mistakes we make in trying to know, of the things that interfere with our knowing, of what we are not interested in and do not really want to know,' (ibid.: 64). In this chapter I elaborate on these types of knowledge for medical professionals, and propose that they become particularly important in efforts to resist commercial investments in clinical evidence by considering the limits to extrapolation from pharmaceutical trials; awareness of the play of chance in individual experiments; and gaps in the evidence base because of trials that cannot or will not be done. I end by suggesting that more might be done to make these issues visible in publishing trials and to connect such collective critique with the original educational agenda of EBM.

Policing the RCT and Tackling Corporate Science

Suspicion of commercially sponsored research is nothing new. In the 1950s the methodological rigour of randomisation, blinding and other refinements of clinical experimentation was proposed to discipline industry's investigations and claims (Marks, 2002). Yet as industry adopted the basic framework of the RCT, more subtle distortions of the evidence have become apparent to clinical scientists, who have been at the forefront of efforts to respond. One early complaint was about the tendency for negative or inconvenient results to disappear (Sackett, 1979). Described as a form of 'publication bias' (Dickersin, 1990) and a pressing ethical issue (Chalmers, 1990), this problem has led to calls for public registration of trials before and after completion, an approach that has finally gained support from journal editors, the World Health Organisation and the US Food and Drug Administration in recent years, though not all manufacturers.[1]

Other research on commercial trials has described more insidious forms of 'methodological bias.' These include the ability of industry to produce apparently impressive results by choosing inappropriate comparators, patient groups or outcomes for trials of their products (Djulbegovic et al 2001), or using inadequate samples or follow up periods, even ending trials early (Boyd, 2001). We can identify three kinds of responses to these problems, all designed to prevent companies promoting their products at the expense of public health.

The first approach could be labelled 'educational': transmitting skills for what is known as critical appraisal to individual clinicians (e.g. Guyatt et al., 1993). This has evolved from giving doctors basic information about the play of chance in experiments[2] and asking them to look for evidence of appropriate randomisation or blinding, to more sophisticated efforts to represent the magnitude of effect through absolute rather than relative risk reduction (Naylor et al., 1992), and account for the importance of results through calculations of Numbers Needed To Treat (Cook and Sackett, 1995).

The second approach relies on expert work and funding for an additional layer of research characterised by the use of meta-analysis in systematic reviews of the evidence on particular clinical questions. This has become increasingly important thanks to the success of institutions such as the UK's Cochrane Collaboration

---

1   Journal editors claimed to take a lead here in 2005, when members of the International Committee of Medical Journal Editors agreed not to publish unregistered studies. In 2007 the WHO produced standards for such registers and the FDA Amendments Act required registration from clinical trials of medicines and devices subject to FDA regulation.

2   In part by increasing the use of the confidence interval over the p value as a measure of significance.

and has been adopted by many bodies producing guidelines at a national level. According to Moreira (2007) the techniques of systematic review offer a means of 'disentanglement' by which reviewers aim to 'resist the enticements, persuasive strategies and arguments inscribed in papers,' diluting the commercial agendas performed within a single study.

The final approach is 'regulatory' in that it looks to impose reporting standards for trials, to require trial registration and make data publicly available for further scrutiny. Reporting standards are expected to work as 'checks and balances' on commercial science (Chopra, 2003) through checklists such as CONSORT (Begg et al., 1996) that demand adequate information on methodology, as well as standardised reporting of conflicts of interest and authorship. Academic approaches to this issue have recently been supplemented by apparent attempts at self-regulation from industry itself (Graf et al., 2009).

All these strategies tend to filter out key elements of trials to achieve greater clarity about their message and importance for clinical practice. There is some irony that the concerns about industry influence often appear alongside evidence of the lack of impact of research evidence on practice. Yet in the case of new drugs, the money spent on orders for large numbers of 'off-prints' of journal articles for distribution to prescribers, suggest that industry is convinced that these can influence doctors' decisions. Responding to this marketing activity, some social scientists argue that professional and regulatory strategies are still not enough to tackle the ways in which trials carry commercial interests into the clinic.

For Sismondo (2009) industry funded trials are a form of 'corporate science' – investigations that are designed to look like academic work but actually further marketing messages. This argument builds on earlier accounts of trials as experimental in a broader sense, a means for companies and clinicians to settle on a precise clinical indication for which a new drug may be marketed (Oudshoorn, 1993). Detailed empirical studies suggest that research creates markets by establishing new conditions or expanding the indications for pharmaceutical treatment, as well as building up professionals who can act as spokespeople for the product (Fishman, 2004; Rasmussen, 2004; 2005; Sismondo, 2009). The very design of trials contains commercial agendas (Sismondo, 2008) by shifting scientific and clinical attention and producing blueprints for new protocols (Will, 2009).

This connection between trials and commercial 'agenda setting' is hard to tackle. Systematic review, accompanied by increased trial registration, has an important role in identifying the full set of trials on a particular question, and areas of uncertainty, but will inevitably give most visibility to areas where trials have been done. It has been suggested that the best response would be to ask journals to stop publishing articles that are commercially sponsored and provide public funding for trials (Doucet and Sismondo, 2008), but this significant regulatory step looks unlikely for the present. This chapter focuses instead on attempts to strengthen critical appraisal through journals as the site where most clinicians first encounter trial data.

Professional Reflection as a Resource for the Ethnographer

As discussed above, many clinical scientists understand these issues and are working to find solutions. The material that informs my analysis reflects more than five years sustained engagement with such researchers and guideline writers in the area of cardiovascular disease. In seeking to contribute to efforts to think about evidence in medicine, I follow Holmes and Marcus (2006) in attempting to 'work within and through domains of representation and practice' of experts, using their reflection as a source, a kind of 'para-ethnography' of a field.

This field is delineated here by the publication of research on a drug called rosuvastatin. Statins are a class of drugs marketed as a means of lowering low-density lipoprotein (LDL) (often referred to more simply as cholesterol) and thereby reducing the risk of heart disease. The first statins were used in the 1980s and sales swelled throughout the 1990s. However, in launching rosuvastatin (TM Crestor) in 2003 AstraZeneca claimed that it was stronger that existing statins and had additional positive effects. Their campaign gained unwelcome attention when an Editorial in *The Lancet* attacked the company for endangering public health by 'blatant marketing dressed up as research' (Horton, 2003a: 1341). He argued that they had not yet produced convincing evidence for their claims for rosuvastatin and that statements by prominent clinicians about its value were misleading. Below I will provide a closer analysis of this rather unusual intervention, before investigating the publication of other rosuvastatin data to explore the broader presentation of trial evidence in journals. A more theoretical discussion will then draw out some of the epistemic strategies used by contemporary editors to guide readings of these trials, making contextual information, and, critically, 'negative knowledge' visible to a clinical audience.

An Editor's Attack on Some 'Adventurous Statistics'

Horton's Editorial appeared five months after rosuvastatin was first marketed in the UK. The drug was entering a crowded market and the company was said to have set aside the largest marketing budget for a single product in history. *The Lancet*'s editor was unimpressed complaining that promotional material raised 'disturbing questions about how drugs enter clinical practice and what measures exist to protect patients from inadequately investigated medicines,' (Horton, 2003a: 1341). In making this argument, he referred both to information about the commercial context for the launch and methodological failings in the published data.

Commercial Information

Horton started with an unusual personal attack on the Managing Director of AstraZeneca, and reference to falls in the company's pre-tax profits. A really critical reading of the evidence on rosuvastatin, he implied, depended on understanding the precariousness of AstraZeneca's share price and intense competition between different statins, some of which were coming off patent. Though the title of the piece designated it as part of 'the statin wars' – a term that had also been used to refer to fierce competition between the new drug and those already on the market, especially Merck Sharp and Dohme's (MSD) simvastatin and Pfizer's atorvastatin, Horton acknowledged this only obliquely, suggesting that doctors should not use the new product given the existence of older products with more extensive efficacy and safety data.

The Limits of Extrapolation

Horton then turned to the quality of the evidence offered to doctors. The company presented its research on rosuvastatin as part of an interlinked set of trials, under the title GALAXY. This appeared to give breadth to the evidence for the drug, but there was no detailed information on every study. In his Editorial Horton focussed his attack on a lack of depth in the programme, based on trials that were in the public domain. Though these appeared to have adhered to the basic methodological standards that give credibility to the RCT, it was dangerous to extrapolate from these to medical practice.

The first trial, STELLAR, was a study of more than 2000 patients, published in a peer-reviewed journal in 2002. Horton argued that follow-up in this study was too short, averaging six weeks, and more importantly that it was inappropriate to use cholesterol levels as endpoints, rather than the 'clinical' issues of mortality or morbidity (heart attacks, strokes etc.). A second publication – this time published only in a promotional supplement to a journal – combined results from a number of similarly brief trials. Making no reference to the activities of regulators who had approved the drug for sale, Horton argued that trials of rosuvastatin needed to be longer and measure mortality in order to convince doctors of the drug's safety.

The Adequacy of Surrogate Endpoints

By dismissing both LDL cholesterol and measures of vessel thickness as 'soft endpoints' Horton countered the company's message that 'the lower the cholesterol, the better' for the patient. This agenda was built around rosuvastatin's ability to reduce cholesterol by greater amounts than other statins. Horton's imagined reader appeared to be the individual clinician, who was susceptible to the excitement surrounding a new drug launch. He did not acknowledge the fact that surrogate endpoints might represent a compromise between regulators and manufacturers or researchers, as has happened in both AIDS research and oncology (Epstein, 1997, Keating and Cambrosio, 2003). Rather by rejecting 'surrogate' endpoints for those he called 'clinical' – especially mortality – Horton appeared to ask the reader to make an independent judgement about the value of cholesterol levels in this case.[3]

Horton's intervention can be contrasted with other efforts to encourage critical appraisal of endpoints in commercial drug trials. A popular series in the BMJ in the 1990s ('How to read a paper') had focussed on this question specifically. Like Horton, Greenhalgh (1997) distinguished between outcomes 'that matter to patients' (the progression of disease or illness, reassurance, palliation etc.) and the 'targets' of treatment. These targets might be physiological markers such as cholesterol, but the author reminded readers that they needed to be related to patient care. Unlike Horton, she offered ways to judge their appropriateness by tracking the chronological connections between movements in the markers and in disease for populations or individuals, or agreeing on a logical connection based on evidence that the markers and clinical outcomes varied together in both directions, demonstrated a dose response relationship *and* could be linked to a biologically plausible explanation.

In Greenhalgh's schema, the clinical reader needed to bring together different forms of expertise to sustain an appropriately critical appraisal of a paper. Physiological and pharmacological understanding might inform a judgement about the value of surrogates and careful extrapolation from published studies. Practical experience should give the ability to identify outcomes important to patients. In his Editorial Horton added a further category of knowledge, referring to the commercial context for this particular launch. What are the chances that this depth of appraisal could be achieved for any particular paper? In the next section I consider the role of editorials in guiding interpretation of a subsequent mortality trial of rosuvastatin, JUPITER, to illustrate ways in which *The Lancet* and other journals have attempted to produce this kind of critique.

Editorials as Public Appraisal

Despite the bitterness of Horton's attack in 2003, in April 2009, rosuvastatin investigators published a paper coming out of the JUPITER data in the journal. Though presented as an exploratory, rather than experimental study, driven by academic interest, this piece clearly fitted with the company's interest in setting a particular agenda around statin use: an emphasis on magnitude of cholesterol reduction, supporting the use of 'more potent statins' and the use of a dual target (LDL cholesterol *and* C-reactive protein (CRP) as an inflammatory marker for heart disease).

---

3   This is not the insistence on mortality as most easily standardised/measured endpoint in large, multi-centred clinical trials. Instead Horton draws on an important further strand of EBM, which insists that only mortality expresses a suitably 'modest' position for medicine as a possible source of unintended harms.

This time Horton made no personal intervention. Instead two commissioned editorials were published alongside the paper arguing that the data should be treated with some scepticism. Rather than focus on market information, or problems of extrapolation from surrogate endpoints, the authors modelled forms of critique grounded in the gap between research and practice and the play of chance in experimental research. These arguments were framed by statements of potential 'conflicts of interest'. All the authors of the first piece had received research money from rosuvastatin's manufacturers, and the lead writer was actively involved in a mortality trial of rosuvastatin at the time of writing. This was characterised carefully as 'investigator initiated, funded by Canadian Institutes for Health Research and AstraZeneca' (Yusuf et al., 2009). The author of the second commentary was a cardiologist who acknowledged that he had been a speaker or sat on advisory boards for a wide range of pharmaceutical companies, including AstraZeneca and their competitors, Pfizer, MSD and Novartis (Despres, 2009).

The Limits of a Single Study

Despite these interests, both commentaries reflected on the JUPITER trial to express doubts about treatment at lower levels of LDL or high CRP. Despres argued that the study was of more scientific than practical interest, offering a proof of the concept that reducing CRP *might* reduce cardiovascular events.

> From a pathophysiological standpoint, JUPITER provides key experimental data that inflammation is an important mediator of the clinical benefits of rosuvastatin. However, to immediately translate these findings into clinical practice without appropriate and careful discussion of their implications is not prudent (Despres, 2009: 1148).

This statement made the trial a way of probing a particular narrative about the workings of the body, 'experimental' in a broader sense than a single comparison between two forms of treatment. The implications were complicated enough to require 'careful discussion' over time.

In a second Editorial Yusuf and co-authors struck a still more negative note by setting reports of two other trials alongside that of JUPITER to case doubt on the arguments being made by the investigators. CORONA and GISSI had also lowered vascular events and mortality, but in CORONA having a high CRP had been no barrier to experiencing this benefit (Yusuf et al., 2009). JUPITER cardiovascular mortality gains were also greater than would be predicted from the cholesterol reductions in other studies. The very strong mortality advantage for rosuvastatin in JUPITER appeared to them as 'excessive': lower rates of death from cancer in the intervention groups were 'not biologically plausible' (average follow up was too short to see an effect on cancer), so 'chance might have exaggerated the apparent benefits in JUPITER (compounded by the trial's early termination)' (ibid.: 1154).

Alternative Knowledge

Both commentaries focussed on the possibilities of the trial as evidence for narratives about the pathophysiology underlying cholesterol control. Here it appeared that expert commentary was properly concerned with discussion of mechanism, rather than the headline results, drawing some distance between both considerations and the decision to change clinical practice. As in other cases, physiological reasoning is constantly invoked in the work of trial interpretation (Will, 2009).

The effect of such expert contributions on the ordinary reader is inevitably hard to judge. However, correspondence around the study report followed the pattern of introducing alternative sources of knowledge to challenge the proposal that rosuvastatin should be used to lower LDL and CRP together. Strikingly, these letters reproduced Greenhalgh's (1997) arguments about the use of surrogates. For example, one used the existence of people with genetically high levels of CRP but no apparent increased risk of vascular disease to add to doubts about the link between the marker and morbidity (Garcia de Tena, 2009). Another suggested that elevated CRP was itself a 'surrogate' for other lipid changes: 'the use of HDL cholesterol instead of CRP is on much firmer grounds pathophysiologically' (Feeman, 2009: 24). Others questioned the scope of the data: no continuous relationship had been demonstrated between CRP and risk/benefit (Sniderman, 2009); the trialists had not modelled the practice they proposed either by increasing the dose to reach specific targets of CRP or cholesterol (Rosenstein and Parra, 2009), or responding to CRP levels specifically (Danchin, 2009).

The effectiveness of correspondence in raising questions about extrapolation to clinical practice appeared to offer some support to Horton's own beliefs in this genre – which he had previously discussed as part of the 'post publication review process' (Horton, 2002). Writing in JAMA, he argued then that 'research reports leave deep critical footprints in the medical literature', but that all too often authors failed to respond to readers' letters, and that subsequent guidelines were not informed by such collective appraisal. His solution, perhaps illustrated by the presence of two separate articles in 2009, was to continue to explore what he called 'pluralist' journal publication. Yet his 2003 Editorial also acknowledged limitations on the ability of experts to produce critical and independent accounts of trial data.

Editorial Voices

Tension Between Eminence and Evidence

EBM has traditionally been sceptical about the authority claimed by experts (eminence) rather than given to trial data, not least because of the potential for both financial and scientific interests to cloud expert judgement. This concern was clearly evident in Horton's 2003 discussion of trials published before JUPITER.

> Based on these tentative surrogate findings, one Stellar investigator, Peter Jones, commented that, 'If I have the option of achieving goals at a lower comparable dose, I would choose that. This kind of gloss does little to foster sensible, let alone critical, appraisal of weak data' (Horton 2003a: 1341).

Researchers in the field were reducing the space for 'critical' readings by individual doctors: those who might be expected to model appraisal had failed to do so. This might also prevent future research. 'Talking up the efficacy of statins subverts efforts to conduct large-scale outcome trials where they matter most – e.g., in heart failure,' (ibid.). This belief in the power of the expert voice appeared somewhat justified given the response to Horton's own intervention. A very high number of downloads from Science Direct resulted in it being the Most Wanted article from the journal in 2003.

In response, AstraZeneca sought to appeal to both 'eminence' and 'evidence,' defending the experts who had recommended the new product and appealing to the authority of regulators who had already accepted the drug's safety. But despite the large number of downloads, relatively few other responses to it were published. One that was picked up on Horton's invocation of the individual clinical decision to suggest that there really was not a problem: doctors could distinguish between commercial or personal interest and good evidence.

> We, as doctors, have the option to accept or reject marketing practices ... If we want more data, we can wait and prescribe when we feel comfortable with the data (if ever). Marketing is not just an AstraZeneca issue, and personal attacks on an individual or a product is [sic] not the solution (Wozniak 2003: 1855).

This response suggested that individual practitioners were capable of their making their own critical readings, and acting upon them. At the same time, it made Horton's 'personal attacks' suspect.[4] In fact another correspondent 'invited' Horton to make his own conflict of interest statement hinting that there was a risk that he was somehow himself involved in the battle between different statins (Kernick, 2003).

Accounting for Personal and Institutional Interest

Though conflict of interest statements have been common practice in major journals since the late 1990s, Horton himself had previously expressed doubts about their value. Cautioning against a belief that any scientific report could be truly objective because of their inherently rhetorical nature, he argued then that it was not clear how people should interpret a statement of interest that simply followed the report, and that narrow financial statements did not capture the full

---

4   See McGoey 2009 for other cases where individual interventions have been portrayed as suspect in comparison with apparently impersonal appeals to the data.

range of involvements that might lie behind authorship (Horton, 1997). His own statement following publication of the 2003 Editorial did, however, focus on the financial aspect.

> If a company withdrew its advertising or stopped buying reprints from *The Lancet*—for example, if we published a piece critical of their marketing practices—the journal's revenue could fall. A drop in *The Lancet's* income could conceivably diminish my personal remuneration. The business climate for most modern medical journals, whether in the for-profit or non-profit sector, is strongly pro-pharmaceutical industry. The industry is an important and much-valued customer for medical publishers. In this environment, I know that it can be difficult for editors to raise questions about the ethics and marketing tactics of pharmaceutical companies, not only in what we write and publish but also in applying strict advertising guidelines. *The Lancet's* editors have long had, and continue to have, complete editorial independence over decisions concerning content (Horton 2003b: 1856).

Much as in the two pieces cited above, this statement somewhat perversely appeared to give reasons why Horton might not have written the piece – *increasing* the sense that it was a disinterested intervention. The statement did not mention the publicity for the journal attendant on his attack, and the way in which it positioned journals on the side of patient safety against corporate greed. Instead it echoed his Editorial in offering information about the commercial context for clinical research and publication. Journals continue to struggle with the facts of their own interest, as well as the difficulty of finding any expert to offer commentary who has not at some point taken money from pharmaceutical companies in order to carry out research.

Collective Critique?

One way to respond to this problem might be to further increase the number of voices speaking on any particular issue, diluting partisan comment in much the same way as meta-analysis dilutes the impact of an individual trial. An illustration of this approach can be found in editorial strategies surrounding the publication of the main JUPITER trial in the *New England Journal of Medicine*. Results from the commercially funded study came out in 2008, apparently offering the mortality data that Horton had demanded five years earlier. The trial had enrolled nearly 18,000 people without heart disease who had 'low' cholesterol by contemporary standards, but high levels of C-reactive protein. It was ended early after the data and safety monitoring board noted a significant reduction in the cardiovascular events in the intervention group, and a trend in this direction for heart attacks, stroke and death from cardiovascular causes. However, a number of interventions published alongside the results again struck a sceptical note about the importance of these results for clinical practice.

Modelling Appraisal

The author of the NEJM Editorial addressing the rosuvastatin results claimed to have no financial interest in debates about the drug, and was not a member of the NEJM board. Indeed he started with his doubts about the use of drugs in prevention.

> The aphorism 'prevention is better than cure' makes perfect sense when applied to healthy habits such as following a sensible diet, maintaining an ideal body weight, exercising regularly, and not smoking. But increasingly, prevention of cardiovascular disease includes drug therapy, particularly statins to lower cholesterol levels ... Before pharmacological treatment for primary prevention is expanded further, however, the evidence should be examined critically (Hlatky, 2008: 2280).

In the remainder of the article Hlatky went on to model his version of critical appraisal. First he summarised the JUPITER trial according to trial population, follow up, endpoints and outcomes, including confidence intervals: the same strategy as Horton but pursued more systematically. Next he asked two questions, which served to focus his article. 'Should indications for statin treatment be expanded? And how should measurements of high-sensitivity C-reactive protein be used?' His response to the first was negative, informed by reference to absolute rather than relative measures of risk reductions extrapolated from the JUPITER trial, using a key tool of EBM in the Number Needed To Treat.

> The proportion of participants with hard cardiac events in JUPITER was reduced from 1.8% (157 of 8901 subjects) in the placebo group to 0.9% (83 of the 8901 subjects) in the rosuvastatin group; thus, 120 participants were treated for 1.9 years to prevent one event (ibid.).

Hlatky's presentation provided an exceptionally clear statement of the limited benefits of using the drug in the way used in the trial. Given this, like Horton, he was concerned about safety. Rosuvastatin had been associated with raised haemoglobin and diabetes, and the trial did not offer long-term safety data on large reductions in LDL. A third problem lay in the cost compared with off-patent statins.

However, as his initial questions suggested, Hlatky was not only interested in whether rosuvastatin should be used, but also whether statins in general might be useful in people with lower levels of LDL cholesterol than the current thresholds, and whether CRP was a helpful additional measure of risk. Though these questions appeared more general than the value of the individual product, in fact they were central to the marketing of rosuvastatin, since the company had chosen to associate it with efforts to expand the indications for drug treatment in both these areas – the 'agenda-setting' work discussed above. Here Hlatky was again critical, complaining in particular about a lack of fit between the emphasis on CRP and the study in general.

> The trial did not compare subjects with and those without high-sensitivity C-reactive protein measurements, nor did it compare the use of high-sensitivity C-reactive protein with the use of other markers of cardiovascular risk … JUPITER was a trial of statin therapy, not high-sensitivity C-reactive protein testing (ibid.: 2281).

On the face of it then the NEJM piece poured cold water on the company's interest not only in promoting its new drug, but also exerting downward pressure on cholesterol thresholds and adding new measures of risk. The commentary combined detailed reference to the data in a specific trial with a personal view on the most important issues at stake.

Rapid Responses

What might be the effect of such arguments? At the same time as publishing the editorial material and trial report, the NEJM took the more unusual step of opening a poll and a forum for discussion, under the title 'Clinical Directions'. This approach had some similarity with the use of rapid responses online by the BMJ (from which a smaller number of letters are selected for print publication). Would these editorial strategies improve the 'quality of debate'? And what would they suggest about the effects of the paper and the Editorial as opposing testimonials about the value of rosuvastatin?

As students of the trend for public consultation on scientific questions have repeatedly pointed out, the poll is a very minimal form of involvement, reducing complex issues to propositional questions. In this case the journal asked two things of its readers:

> Do you believe, on the basis of the JUPITER trial results, that the approach to laboratory screening of apparently healthy adults should be changed? [and] Do you believe, on the basis of the JUPITER trial results, that the therapeutic use of statins in apparently healthy adults should be changed? (NEJM, 2009).

The results suggested a fairly even split between accepting the company's interpretation of the results and the more critical Editorial (51% against shifts in laboratory screening; 52% against greater use of statins). Though the NEJM poll appeared to gain some authority by the sheer numbers of responses received: 'over 18 days, 2553 people voted,' (Kritek and Campion, 2009), the journal's editors made little comment about this split in opinion.

An equally mixed response was seen in qualitative responses to an online forum set up to appear alongside the trial report in the internet version. This garnered a lower level of participation: approximately 470 responses (of which 85% came from practicing physicians, 20% from cardiologists), but the range of actual comments made it more interesting. In particular, of those who were doubtful about the value of JUPITER, many quoted numbers needed to treat from the trial like Hlatky, while others echoed his concern with cost, diabetes and the study's early termination. Other than briefly citing these issues, the journal made no further efforts to analyse the responses however, apart from thanking those who 'took time to post comments for others to read,' (Kritek and Campion, 2009). The editors did not, for example, distil original points for further discussion.

The NEJM's experiments with both poll and forum appeared to add little to an expert commentary, which set the agenda for critique, simply appearing alongside commercially funded studies as a kind of counter balance. Indeed, though sharing Hlatky's interest in the NNT as a key absence from the JUPITER report, posts to the forum did not offer the same kind of careful analysis of gaps in the evidence base. The propositional format favoured a focus on action rather than reflection, asking doctors what they would 'do' rather than exploring what they felt they knew or took to be areas of uncertainty.

The Role of Journals: Working with Corporate Data

Journals are still a key site where different groups come together to settle what will be allowed to count as data in the clinical context. It could be argued that these efforts to produce Horton's 'cultures of critique' (2002) are ultimately irrelevant. As *The Lancet* editor argued then, even published challenges to trials may not inform guidelines, and there is evidence that trial results have a limited effect on prescribing decisions made by individual clinicians. Yet there remains the problem of the agenda setting work of trials, which may have more insidious effects on medical practice. Trial registration offers one way to control the company's interest in 'spinning' the evidence to fit current marketing messages, asking authors to demonstrate fidelity to a previously published protocol. Yet it may also add to the power of this protocol as a vehicle for commercial agendas, such as creating or expanding indications for drug treatment. This dimension of commercial studies is a real challenge for journal editors if they restrict themselves to commenting only on 'scientific' aspects of a study.

The examples given in this chapter help illustrate the use of editorial material, traditional letters and innovations such as the readers' poll to bring commercially funded trials into question, identifying problems and gaps remaining after the publication of trial outcomes. What can we say about the epistemic culture within which these genres emerge? What sense can be made theoretically of the 'data work' performed through them, and relationships established between different ways of knowing in journals?

Negative Knowledge and the Work of Elaboration

At the start of this chapter I noted that attempts to standardise trial reporting, and produce systematic reviews of multiple studies, rely on work to filter out the key points from data that has been brought into existence through the RCT. This has the potential to create positive knowledge by giving trial results credibility within the medical community. Yet EBM might also be seen as a set of techniques for managing and making visible clinical uncertainty.[5] In this chapter, I have drawn out a number of possible sources of this uncertainty. The challenge for journals is to find ways of acknowledging these as relevant for the project of collective appraisal. Though at first view, the experiments in high-energy physics, described by Knorr Cetina (1999), look very different from the clinical trials discussed in this collection, her analysis of 'negative knowledge' is suggestive of ways to think about uncertainty remaining after trial data is available. Here I draw out some of these issues for medicine, using Knorr Cetina's three-part typology.

Limits of knowing   This first category is particularly important for medicine, not least to inform priorities for future clinical research. When viewed as a problem for the individual trial, uncertainty emerges around the problem of extrapolation. Complaints about surrogate endpoints and length of follow up in experiments on groups of patients draw force from concerns about the potential for medicine to cause unintended harms, perhaps by mechanisms that are not well understood. In critiquing trials, the Number Needed To Treat calculation emerges as a particularly powerful means of setting out the uncertain benefits of preventive treatment for individuals. Here a 'modest' EBM gives doctors not only means of producing positive information, but also of elaborating on the limits of knowing.

Mistakes in trying to know   The second category is also acknowledged by careful reports on the meaning of trial data, especially the possible play of chance in any single study. In my examples this emerged in doubts about the mortality benefits attributed to rosuvastatin. In making this argument, both Despres and Yusuf et al also drew on additional forms of medical knowledge (Tanenbaum, 1994), notably physiology, to supplement trial results and attempt to judge their significance. For Yusuf et al., variations and inconsistencies between studies should not be smoothed out but made the subject of further reflection. Where Horton viewed a patho-physiological argument with suspicion in the hands of industry, clinical experts could also use it to challenge the value of an individual, and rather expensive, product.[6]

---

5   Chalmers, May 2008, personal communication.

6   This can also be seen as a late expression of the tensions held together in the trial itself, for expert researchers generally take on studies out of an interest in these physiological processes which form the currency of specialist academic research, while companies are focussed on the effects on groups of patients by Phase III trials.

Interferences with knowing The final category of negative knowledge that emerged in this chapter related to economic and institution reasons for gaps in the evidence base, and information about the commercial context. The notion of trials not done was important in nearly all attempts at appraisal. Often this led to calls for alternative trials in the future. More strikingly, however, Hlatky's Editorial also reminded the reader that many trials would never be funded – invoking the importance of lifestyle change as an alternative to drugs in prevention.

Another warning to the clinical reader related more specifically to the commercial context for research. The classic example here is the conflict of interest statement, which elaborates on the financial and professional involvement of the author in the production of evidence. As Horton himself pointed out however (1997), it is often unclear how such information should be understood. In the case of rosuvastatin, editors used their involvement in other trials, or other work for pharmaceutical companies, to provide evidence of their expertise and disinterest, as much as markers for potential bias. Though EBM has drawn 'eminence' into question as a source of knowledge, expert voices continue to be important sources of critical views for journals, and acquire authority because of rather than despite involvement in research, including commercial-funded studies.

Horton's 2003 Editorial was less typical in offering doctors information about pressure on AstraZeneca's share price at the time of the rosuvastatin launch, and the size of the marketing budget. This information is difficult for journals to manage because it is so linked to the moment of publication. However it appeared to find an enthusiastic audience. The problem for attempts to make readers aware of this context is that the precise effects have to be inferred, the scope of the methodological bias hinted at is often not identified. As with the conflict of interest statement, this information does not say directly whether editorial messages should be discounted or accepted in their entirety, or which aspects of their intervention are more or less compromised. In that sense they offer 'ignorance' as much as knowledge, but are no less suggestive of the need for caution about the results of the commercial trial.

The Importance of Ignorance

The types of critique examined in this chapter appear rather different from the strategies of those carrying out systematic reviews or working to standardise trial reporting, proceeding by elaboration and contextualisation rather than filtration of evidence. Both Editorials and letters offered accounts of negative knowledge and ignorance to clinical readers alongside positive claims in trial reports. McGoey (2007) has argued that claims of ignorance are a powerful weapon in the hands of regulators and pharmaceutical companies, who use them to resist questions about the safety of a particular drug in widespread use. Here discussions of ignorance emerge as important elements of the *professional* appraisal of commercial trials. Thus trial data may be framed by references to other epistemic traditions in medicine, and both expert and generalist views may be granted brief personal authority in order to make these interventions.

The effectiveness of these strategies is unclear: the NEJM poll offers only the vaguest evidence of their possible ability to confuse. However, it seems reasonable to briefly imagine oneself a reader and consider what one might make of the Editorial, letters, poll or forum as addenda to the trial report. Here Horton's earlier critique of the conflict of interest statement appears pertinent. Reporting conventions as developed in journals to date, bring a myriad of different interests into view, but do not contain any attempt to sum up the likely results.

Conclusion

Each commercially funded trial is an experiment in how to hold different interests in balance: not only corporate science versus academic investigation, but also the concerns of payers with costs, governments with innovation; the careers of professional researchers, and patients' desire for care or treatment. Journals appear to bring their own interest in accessing trials as marketable information and sustaining relationships with commercial actors who provide a good deal of their funding. However, they act in more complicated ways than this would suggest, thanks to the power of cultural and professional investments in the idea of peer review, the professional community and public health. The question is how far they can still act as a resource for those seeking to promote good patient care.

In this chapter I have focussed less on publication bias, than on the potential for methodological bias and further 'agenda-setting' work in commercially sponsored trials. EBM's original focus on critical appraisal remains important if doctors are to resist these pressures. Its individual focus, however, may represent a significant limit. Only some doctors will choose to go on further training, and there are doubts about the effectiveness of workshops for giving doctors skills and inculcating sceptical attitudes to the evidence, even when it comes in the form of the RCT. Creating spaces for debate and sharing responses to trials appear to offer an interesting way of making trial appraisal a collective project.

The problem for editors is finding ways of activating diverse information and professional opinion. In this case, the authority of numbers associated with individual trials was repeatedly challenged by expert voices drawing on other trials, patho-physiological knowledge and information about the organisation of industry, financial markets and health care. Strikingly in this case, such voices appeared to gain, rather than lose, credibility by virtue of their 'interestedness'. Though efforts to involve a broader professional public in the discussion appear fashionable, it is tempting to argue that working through key areas of 'negative knowledge' is a more important task for journals than the efforts to generate debate for its own sake. There may however be more to do to elaborate on the different forms of negative knowledge, or uncertainty, balancing the power of the visible results from individual trials or sets of studies, including those funded by industry, with awareness of the trials not done and the questions unanswered.

Chapter 5

When are Trials Not Enough?
Clinical Versus Cost-effectiveness in the
Controversy Over Access to
Dementia Drugs in the NHS

Tiago Moreira

Whither Clinical Effectiveness?

In the past two decades, the epistemic authority of clinical trials has suffered significant challenges. Developed in the mid years of the 20th century as a methodological device to ascertain the effects of therapeutics above and beyond those that come from clinical empathy or marketing persuasion, the randomised controlled clinical trial (RCT) has been key mediator in the relationships and tensions between therapeutic developers, regulators, epidemiologists, clinicians, patients, political stakeholders and a variety of publics (Marks, 1997). With the institutionalisation, in the second half of the last century, of the requirement to demonstrate clinical efficacy in order to obtain therapeutic marketing licences in the United States and Europe, the RCT became an integral part of drug research and development. By the end of the century, however, a variety of critiques emerged that questioned whether the RCT was still able to secure the public health of nations and communities (see Introduction). In this chapter, I take what we called the 'economic critique' as my point of departure, particularly its claim that a) clinical trials and the ideal of clinical effectiveness do not provide a good enough basis to make decisions about how to produce health in society and b) new tools need to be used to ascertain cost-effectiveness and opportunity costs derived from resource allocation scenarios.

The aim of the chapter is to analyse how, when and for whom cost-effectiveness can be said to be more important that clinical effectiveness. In the background is the establishment, in the past 15 years, of different systems of priority setting or 'explicit rationing' of health care in a variety of countries (Ham and Roberts, 2003). In the United Kingdom, this policy has been embodied in the workings of the National Institute of Clinical Excellence or NICE (now National Institute for Health and Clinical Excellence), a Special Health Authority within the National Health Service (NHS) created in 1999 to provide professionals and patients with standards of health care based on the best available evidence. NICE is distinctive in that it specifically uses cost-utility analysis and Quality Adjusted Life Years (QALY) to frame its guidance on cost – as well as clinical – effectiveness of groups of technologies. Clinical effectiveness as demonstrated by RCTS is not enough. As Rawlins and Culyer, two of the institutional designers of NICE put it in the BMJ:

> On its own, clinical effectiveness is insufficient for maintaining or introducing any clinical procedure or process. Cost must also be taken into account. When good evidence exists of the therapeutic equivalence between two or more clinical management strategies the cheaper option is preferred [...] However, in most instances NICE is confronted with a clinical management strategy that is better than current standard practice but which costs more. NICE must then decide what increase in health (compared with standard practice) is likely to accrue from the increase in expenditure. This is the incremental cost effectiveness ratio. Such ratios can be expressed in many ways. NICE's preferred measure is the cost per quality adjusted life year (Rawlins and Culyer, 2004: 224).

NICE's preference for cost-effective assessments above and beyond clinical effectiveness is underpinned by a significant shift in the political understanding of the health care provided within the NHS. Where the ideal was once to provide health care according to need, the requirement is now for commissioning bodies such as Primary Care Trusts to balance assessments of relative need with estimations of the amount of health that is produced by different therapies. The political meaning of this shift is revealed most acutely in the public controversies that have arisen about NICE's advice not to fund therapies for conditions such as multiple sclerosis, kidney cancer, liver cancer and dementia. In all of these conflicts, opponents of NICE argue that clinically effective treatments should not be denied to patients for whom this treatment might be the only chance to extend their life.

Health economists tend to interpret these arguments as understandable grievances which, nonetheless, represent the unavoidable cost of implementing a systematic approach to health care rationing. In this chapter, I wish to take these grievances and arguments seriously. Drawing on the large body of scholarship about scientific and technical controversies (Shapin and Schaffer, 1985; Rip, 1986; Latour, 1987; Callon et al., 2001), the chapter addresses three issues: a) how actors attempt to deconstruct the claim that clinical trials' results and assessments of clinical effectiveness are 'insufficient for maintaining or introducing any clinical procedure or process'; b) how these attempts are, in turn, countered, and by whom; and c) how, through this process, the identities of actors involved in the controversy, their forms of reasoning and the instruments that support them are transformed. For these purposes, I focus on a particular controversy about the use of cost-utility analysis: the public and technical debates surrounding NICE's guidance on access to dementia drugs on the NHS between 2005 and 2007. The chapter is based on a documentary analysis of publicly available materials produced during the controversy, from the technical and policy documents and statements produced by NICE and stakeholders, to reports, articles and editorial pieces published by professional and mainstream media and verbatim transcripts of NICE's appeal hearings obtained by the author under the Freedom of Information Act.

Of particular significance in the analysis presented in this chapter is the changing relationship between knowledge claims presented by NICE and those advanced by the clinical constituency. If, in the beginning of the controversy in 2005, clinicians focused on unpicking the epistemic uncertainties and political entanglements of the QALY as applied to dementia drugs, NICE's 2006 revised advice to fund drugs 'as options in the management of people with Alzheimer's disease of moderate severity only' (NICE, 2006) led opposing sides to explore the relationship between knowledge and political process in health care rationing. Through discussions on NICE's suggestion that the Mini Mental State Examination (MMSE) – a commonly used cognitive test in dementia screening – should be used as a rationing tool, NICE revealed itself as closer to a regulatory, convention-based view of objectivity (Cambrosio et al., 2006) while clinical groups aligned with a mechanical version of objectivity (Daston and Galison, 2007) and criticised NICE's view as a 'technocratic' construct. The subsequent withdrawal of clinicians from public confrontation with NICE can be explained by the way in which these versions of objectivity were seen to belong to different realms of accountability: the public arena, where the MMSE and the QALY embodied the reasonableness and rigour of health care rationing, and the clinical encounter, where the limits of the QALY and the imprecise nature of the MMSE were paradoxically deployed as fundamental to professional practice. This sparks questions about the role of clinical effectiveness in the shifting politics of health care systems and about the way in which such institutional divisions of accountability might be hindering the deployment of new understandings of the role of knowledge in health care.

Modelling the Cost-Utility of Dementia Drugs

Although NICE is required to review its technology appraisals (TA) regularly, in its first review of Alzheimer's disease drugs in 2001 (TA19) it had already recognised that emerging research concerning the cost-effectiveness of these treatments would need to be taken in consideration as soon as possible. TA19 had recommended cholinesterase inhibitors for treatment of mild and moderate dementia mainly on the basis of their clinical effectiveness alone, as the authors considered that the available quality of life measures for dementia had not been validated and judgments on this domain remained uncertain (NICE, 2001). While the overall assessment for clinical effectiveness of cholinesterase inhibitors remained virtually the same over the next few years – that these treatments have modest effects on cognition and are less effective on 'global' clinical measures – the view on the health economics front was changing: it was becoming increasingly accepted that these drugs should be regarded as cost neutral at best, or not cost effective at all.

It was against this backdrop that the Southampton Health Technology Assessment Centre (SHTAC), the research institution commissioned by NICE to carry out a new review, framed its evaluation of dementia treatments. SHTAC researchers drew on the shift in the economic evaluation of these drugs to propose a break with the previous technology appraisal. While they agreed with the argument that most quality of life instruments used in dementia are inadequate and problematic, they suggested, based on a cross-sectional study, that it was possible to draw equivalences between cognitive scores and other dimensions of quality of life to construct 'health utilities' (Loveman et al., 2005). This allowed the SHTAC team to construct an economic model through which they could calculate the cost-per-QALY gained, as the preferred metric used by NICE in their advice to the Department of Health.

SHTAC's model was underpinned by the question: can these treatments delay institutionalisation? It measured the costs of maintaining individuals with dementia in the community with and without treatment (plus cost of care in this health state for the NHS and social services) against the cost of full time care. To be able to construct this model it was essential that 'health states' before and after institutionalisation could be mapped onto data of clinical effectiveness of these drugs. This was because in the absence of clinical trial data on cost-utility (and having rejected the manufacturers' submission on cost-effectiveness) they needed to link the effects of drugs on cognition measures in trials with assumed changes in health utility scores. This led to a calculation of the cost-per-QALY-gained for these treatments of more than two times the NICE's recommended threshold of £35,000 (Rawlins and Culyer, 2004).

Unpicking the Model

Almost immediately after the publication of the draft guidance by NICE, patient organisations, professional organisations and manufacturers publicly aligned in opposition to the advice. The politics of NICE's guidance resonated wide, with newspapers, websites and blogs regularly reporting on these concerns and some linking the response of political representatives to the then upcoming May elections. This was complemented by 'lobbying' MPs in the House of Commons, who brought the issue forward a few weeks later in questions addressed to the then Health Minister Stephen Ladyman.

While the arguments against NICE draft recommendation articulated by the Alzheimer's Society focused on the inadequacy of cognitive measurements and the caring externalities of the economic model, clinicians' criticisms were aimed at the flawed assumptions underpinning the economic model, proceeding by unpicking the uncertainties and ambiguities of measuring quality of life in dementia. A few days after NICE advice was published, the Royal College of Psychiatrists' Faculty of Old Age Psychiatry (RCP/OAP) declared:

We are all very concerned by the implications for our patients of this new advice. In this consultation paper NICE seems to have adopted an inconsistent and contradictory approach that bears little resemblance to the guidance they issued in 2001. NICE agrees that the drugs currently used to treat AD are clinically effective. But the evidence on which they conclude that such drugs are not cost effective is, we strongly believe, flawed (in Irving, 2005).

Similarly, in a letter sent to British Medical Journal on the 15th March 2005, a group of well known old-age psychiatrists argued that,

NICE do not question the safety and efficacy of these drugs but, on a model of cost effectiveness, they conclude that the drugs have failed to meet the level which would justify their prescription on the NHS. However, the model used is largely based on measures that do not have validity in Alzheimer's disease and did not take into account the effects of the disease on carers nor the specific positive benefits of the medications on psychiatric symptoms and behavioural disturbances. The assessment of quality of life in Alzheimer's disease and its economic equivalent quality of life years (QALY's) is not well developed, the model does not do justice to the myriad aspects of the disease and insufficient data are available to support the assumptions presented by NICE. They have carried out a thorough review of the available literature, but what is striking from this is the lack of evidence available on which to base the cost models [...] (Burns et al., 2005).

The argument of clinicians was clear: the validity of the measures used by NICE to construct the QALY concerning dementia drugs was flawed and should not override the valid assessment of clinical effectiveness that NICE itself accepted. The problems relating to measuring quality of life in dementia had been controversial in the field of health technology assessment for a number of years. Clinicians' view was that because most of quality of life instruments in dementia were based on proxy-responders (mainly carers) it was difficult if not impossible to validate such measurements as meaningful assessments of the quality of life of patients. Indeed, it had been on the basis of such assessment that the technology appraisal team had decided not to proceed to an evaluation of health utilities in dementia in 2001. A new appraisal team had come to a different conclusion but, for old age psychiatrists, such measurement remained ambiguous. Later, in the Appeal hearing of July 2006, this argument was made clear by Professor O'Brien on behalf of the RCP/OAP:

In 2001 the appraisal panel looked at the issue of QALYs [...] but they said there were considerable uncertainties and there needed to be another basis for decision-making apart from that. What puzzles us is that the current appraisal with *no new evidence* in the meantime at all on this has taken an entirely different view and taken the QALY to be the primary driver of the decision-making process despite the considerable uncertainties that exist. For example, there is no validated quality of life measure in Alzheimer's Disease. The quality of life measure used in the current appraisal derives from a health utility [instrument] given to a population of US patients with Alzheimer's Disease back in the 1980s and provided utility scores which, when the instrument was revised and compared with a revised version led to significant differences between the two. There is no real consistency there. [...] In that situation we think that other factors should be given more weight, and that has been outlined by Sir Michael Rawlins in the BMJ amongst others when uncertainties exist around the qualities it is important to look at other aspects [...] (Appeal Hearing Transcripts, July 13 2006: 6–7: emphasis added).

Professor O'Brien was attempting to demonstrate that the change in NICE policy *vis-à-vis* QALY for dementia drugs was arbitrary. For this purpose, he highlights that the data used to construct health utilities in SHTAC's model was geographically limited ('population of US patients'), historically contingent ('back in the 1980s') and unreliable ('no real consistency there'). His argument was that NICE's disregard for validity and reliability could not be explained by any account of the pursuit of reason. Recognising uncertainty and avoiding translating it into an action plan should have been the course followed by NICE. In fact, Professor O'Brien argued, NICE's particular advice in this instance appeared to contradict the guidelines provided by its own Chairman Sir Michael Rawlins about how uncertainties should be taken into account when deciding whether or not to use cost-per-QALY-gained measurement. But if NICE's advice could not be 'rationally' understood and contravened its own guidance, what could explain it?

To this question, the clinicians involved in the controversy provided two interlinked answers. Firstly, they argued that NICE's attachment to QALY's was derived from a narrow understanding of quality of life supported by a health economics perspective. As Professor Jones put in the Appeal Hearing 'the whole of this issue is about quality of life, it is not about quality of life years' (37). In asserting this difference, Professor Jones was gesturing towards the particular understanding of quality of life that is contained in the QALY measure. Originally formulated in the United States (Weinstein and Stason, 1977) but since then primarily associated with the University of York (UK), the QALY is underpinned by an 'extra-welfarist' approach to social choice: that is to say that it assumes that maximisation of health, however measured, is the aim of health care systems and that any measurement of health should be equitable and not influenced by willingness to pay (Culyer, 1983; Culyer and Meads, 1992). As a consequence of this, choices should be made on the basis of standardised measurements of health across clinical conditions and therapies. These measurements should also take in consideration aspects of 'utility' that individuals themselves ignore and/or do not value.

According to clinicians, this measurement of quality of life could only be understood as a betrayal of patients' experiences and desires. It was not only that quality of life measurements for dementia were based on other people's views of their lives (see above), but also that such measurements were aimed not at capturing their specific quality of life but at comparing it with other results from patients with other conditions. They thus represented an 'external' view of the needs and 'utilities' of dementia patients. Furthermore, QALY's were based on average effects of therapies and ignored the variability of patient responses, something that had been also recognised in the 2001 NICE guidance. Indeed, one of the clinicians' central criticisms of NICE's 2005 draft guidance was that it had ignored effects that were mostly visible in the consultation room through the relationship between clinician and patient. In the end, clinicians suggested, the desire to have a standardised measurement of health utility had superseded the needs of a specific group of patients and the difficulties with assessing their experiences. Bureaucratic rationality had triumphed over scientific rigour.

Secondly, clinicians articulated the consequences of having so bureaucratic an institution at the heart of the NHS. Already in the letter Professor Burns and colleagues sent to the BMJ, those political meanings were made visible:

> [R]emoval of the anti-dementia drugs will significantly impair our ability to care for people with Alzheimer's disease. [This] will leave private prescriptions the only recourse available to patients and their families to obtain a licensed and proven treatment. This is not only against the ethos of the NHS but leaves vulnerable patients open to the vagaries of the market place (Burns et al., 2005).

The argument presented here is two-fold. For old-age psychiatrists, NICE's decision to rely on inadequate measurements of quality of life would ultimately interfere with the relationship between patient and clinician by withdrawing one of the main material supports of their exchange. The main concern of old-age psychiatrists at this time was that the withdrawal of dementia drugs would undermine the provision of other, care-oriented services that had grown out of the availability of cholinesterase inhibitors. The harmful effects of withdrawing these treatments from the NHS would be felt on various levels, undermining not only services but also the jobs and salaries of those who provide them. It would also be, some argued, a return to the days of therapeutic pessimism and clinical ignorance about dementia. It would be effectively to damage the foundations of a socio-technical world and its way of being.

Out of the ruins of this world another, harsher one would emerge. Patients and families, abandoned to their own devices, would obtain treatment outside the NHS, in the private sector. This would leave 'vulnerable patients open the vagaries of the market place'. By pursuing a technocratic agenda, NICE was effectively ruthlessly forsaking the people who most needed the assistance of the NHS. The political colours of NICE's advice on dementia drugs were now in full view: it was aiming to change the core values of the NHS, its 'ethos'. It was no longer about need but about saving money. Dementia patients were the unfortunate victims of a particular form of technocratic politics.

Linking the Clinic and the Technology Assessment Office?

Such vehement attack on the epistemic, institutional and political foundations of NICE deserved a response. Out of the avalanche of criticism thrown by clinicians, NICE was encouraged by government to take seriously some that pertained to the variability of effectiveness across patient who were given these drugs (Department of Health, 2005). Indeed, one of the clinicians' central criticisms of NICE's draft guidance was that it had ignored patients' variable response to these therapies. Furthermore, while TA19 had recommended that cholinesterase inhibitors should be continued if and while the patient 'responded' to treatment, the new TA111 made no mention of this entity of 'responders'. Sub-group analysis, particularly relating to ambiguous concepts such as 'responders', is a contentious area within medical statistics because of how it might draw on post-randomisation categories to interpret statistical results, especially when these categories were not taken in consideration in 'powering' the study in the first place. There are however specialised statistical techniques that reduce the uncertainty relating to the identification of such groups (Lagakos, 2006). Drawing on this possibility, NICE asked manufacturers to submit further patient level data on such 'responders' and, surprisingly, 'severity of cognition'.

On the 22nd of January 2006, the NICE Appraisals Committee announced its new recommendation that cholinesterase inhibitors should be available on the NHS 'as options in the management of people with Alzheimer's Disease of moderate severity only' (NICE, 2006). This recommendation was underpinned by two decisions: a) not to take into the model the utilities suggested by the Alzheimer's Society, and b) to use 'severity of cognition' as a subgroup rather than 'responders'. In relation to sub-groupings the Committee wrote:

> Overall, the Committee was not persuaded that the responder definition used in TA no. 19, when applied to the results of the pivotal randomised clinical trials, would lead to a cost-effective use of the AChE inhibitors in the NHS.[...] The Committee heard from clinical and patient experts that some people with Alzheimer's disease benefit considerably more from the AChE inhibitors than others, when the results of treatment are analysed retrospectively. It therefore considered whether it might be possible to define, prospectively, subgroups of people with Alzheimer's disease who might benefit more than average, and for whom AChE inhibitors might be a relatively cost-effective treatment (NICE, 2006).

The committee's desire to make the treatments cost-effective appeared here to drive its consideration of the evidence. However rather than using the category of 'responder', their alternative strategy was to explore baseline categories that had been taken into account in the trial size calculations, that is 'prospectively'. As it turned out, it was possible to construct 'sub-groups of people' that were not directly identified in those judgements: defined through severity of cognition. This led to the re-running of the SHTAC model with different utility levels for different 'cognitive' stages of the disease and to the claim that drugs given to patients in the 'moderate' stage of the disease were a good use of public resources. It is important to emphasise this represented an entirely novel way of modelling the relationship between dementia progression and the effects of cholinesterase inhibitors. No equivalent cognition-based claim existed in the literature and, if anything therapeutic developers and evaluators seemed to be suggesting that these drugs should be used as early as possible in order to conserve cognitive abilities (Moreira, 2009). Going against the grain was facilitated by the fact that NICE was publicly framing its guidance as a bridge between what they saw as evidence, on the one hand, and clinical practice, on the other.

A key component of this strategy was the proposal that access to drugs should be mediated by the score obtained by patients in the Mini Mental State Examination (MMSE). Created in 1975 by Folstein and colleagues to assess cognition (Folstein et al., 1975), this tool was conceived as a standardised screening tool that was easy for clinicians to use, and it is regularly used in contemporary practice for this purpose. NICE's proposal was effectively to shift the role of the MMSE from that of a screening tool to a rationing tool: patients would only have access to the drugs if their scores were between 11 and 20 ('moderate'). From NICE's perspective, the MMSE was able to perform this function because it was used in both clinical trials and clinical practice. It represented a settlement between two worlds previously held as incompatible in the controversy. But it was a settlement grounded in the search for cost-effectiveness.

Tools of Partition

NICE's recommendation of January 2006 faced a world that was significantly different from the one encountered by its draft guidance of 2005. While for NICE's consultation process, stakeholders had arranged themselves around two particular issues (see above), in the public sphere, they preferred to present a united front and mobilised to form a public campaign (The Action on Alzheimer's Drugs Alliance). Headed by the Alzheimer's Society, this included professional organisations, other charities and patient organisations, academic institutions and clinical centres. The campaign obtained the support of some national newspapers, most notably the right-wing tabloid the *Daily Mail*. It was also able to call on public support from representatives of the two main parties.

In this context, just two days after NICE issued its second draft guidance, the House of Commons held a hearing with the parties involved in the process. Professor Ballard, an old age psychiatrist, then Head of Research for the

Alzheimer's Society and speaking for the Alliance as a whole attacked the proposal to use the MMSE as a rationing tool with the following statement:

> It is a very useful screening tool. However, a person's score on the test does not equate exactly to the symptoms shown – for example, one person with an MMSE score of 20 might be significantly better at carrying out activities of daily living than another person with the same score. The test is a rough and ready tool. Surely the best way to evaluate the need for drug treatments is the professional judgment of the clinician in consultation with the person and their family. Using the MMSE, it would be extremely easy to score below the desired threshold if people were advised how to do that (Ballard, 2006).

Where NICE had thought of the MMSE as a 'bridge' between trials and the clinic, the Alliance emphasised how, taken in isolation, the MMSE was both an inexact tool and amenable to intentional distortion. The problem again seemed to lie in NICE's misunderstanding of the relationship between standards and clinical practice. The MMSE captured 'roughly' some of the symptoms of dementia; it could only gain meaning through the 'professional judgement of the clinician in consultation with the person and their family'. NICE took what was essentially an 'indicative', heuristic tool and transformed it into something that could discriminate not only between grades of severity of the illness but also between levels of worthiness of patients in prescribing decisions.

The problem was, clinicians argued, that the MMSE scale could not be seen as sensitive to the natural progression of dementia. As one old age psychiatrist put it in a letter to the BMJ:

> MMSE scores do not reflect cognitive decline in dementia in a linear way throughout all the stages of Alzheimer's disease. It is less sensitive to change at each end of its 30-point scale. These drugs will therefore seem to have less of an effect in earlier and later dementia as the MMSE scores at these stages are less sensitive to any change (Molina, 2006).

Clinicians viewed the effects shown on patients with 'moderate dementia' in clinical trials as an effect of the tool rather than an effect of the drug. Because the tool is less sensitive to changes in the earlier and later stages of dementia, 'drugs will therefore seem to have less of an effect' in these stages. But while clinicians understood this and assessed the effects of the drugs in individual patients accordingly, NICE took the instrument and the effects it measured at face value, as a 'black box', ignoring its clinical function and 'inner workings'.

Once again, clinicians provided institutional reasons why such 'black boxing' was possible. NICE's committee and advisors were removed from the clinical relationship and the consultation room. Proposing the MMSE as a rationing tool could only be explained by NICE's exclusion of what the RCP saw as 'relevant clinical expertise': the use of their members as advisors to the Committee, as had happened in 2001. Such exclusion veered NICE towards using inadequate tools and measurements, much in the same way as their decision to use the QALY in their assessment of the effects of dementia drugs (see above). As with the QALY, bureaucratic process had prevailed over a deep and critical understanding of clinical trials.

Both the inadequacy of the QALY in dementia and the issue of the MMSE formed a large part of the appeal clinicians built to contest NICE guidance on the ground of 'perversity'. In alliance with patient organisations and pharmaceutical companies and re-arranging their argument to fit the procedural requirements of the appeals process, clinicians claimed that NICE's guidance was perverse because it advised clinicians to wait until a patient got to a certain level of impairment before treatment could be given. This, they argued, was contrary to reasonable clinical management. Furthermore, reliance on the MMSE to assess cognitive function was a simplification of clinical practice, and would lead to discrimination against groups for which the MMSE was shown to be inadequate (people who were cognitively impaired before contracting dementia and people with English as a second language).

NICE's response was a re-affirmation of their proposed earlier settlement: the MMSE is widely used in clinical trials; it is widely used in clinical practice to express patient progress and thus 'essentially links the evidence to practice' (Professor Stevens in Appeal Hearing Transcript: 130709: 55). But there were changes in their argument. Although not conceding on the issue of the sensitivity of the instrument, for NICE, the fact that it was an imprecise tool was exactly the reason why it had value as a rationing tool in clinical practice.

Epistemically, NICE emphasised the value of the MMSE as a convention. In this, NICE's committee was close to what Cambrosio and colleagues (2006) define as regulatory objectivity. In this version of objectivity, the focus is on the capacity of standards and regulations to mediate between groups and institutions involved in knowledge production and use. Objectivity is convention-based and reliant on workable definitions of problems. Conversely, clinicians favoured a mechanical version of objectivity (Daston and Galison, 2007), which puts the focus on the capacity of representations to adequately mirror phenomena independently of the observer. This tension between versions of objectivity was fundamental to the debate between NICE and clinicians.

The MMSE, NICE appeared to be saying, might not be as 'true' to the nature of dementia as one might wish, but the fact remained that it linked evidence and practice. This however raised questions about why NICE was ready to be so precise about setting score thresholds (11 to 20) with such an imprecise tool:

Chairman: You say that it is soft at the edges and yet you do not give [in the final guidance] any judgement about individual cases […]

Professor Stevens: This gets to the dilemma of whether or not you say: use this but not if you do not want to. We have never really found a solution to that dilemma and I do not think there would be one here either. The guidance is not binding on clinicians. At the end of the day every clinician makes their own judgment about individual cases and that is written in what NICE generally is allowed and is not allowed to do. It is binding on PCTs in terms of funding but it is not absolutely binding. To say, kind of, do not go with it if you do not want to [given that the guidance is not binding] seemed a step too far when in the end what we are charged with is coming up with the best decision we can [...] (Appeal Hearing Transcript: 130709: 56–57).

Here, NICE revealed the political and institutional background to their proposed settlement around MMSE scores. In essence, it was because NICE and the clinicians were doing two different things with the MMSE that it was possible to propose it as link between the clinic and the health technology assessment office. For clinicians, it represented guidance that 'at the end of the day' could be ignored; for NICE, it represented a statement to which they were publicly accountable. There was a 'division of accountability' at work in the process. Clinicians maintained their accountability to individual cases and patients and the basis of this was their clinical autonomy. NICE, on the other hand, saw itself as having to address wider, general concerns about fairness across patients and conditions. As Andrew Dillon, the Chief Executive of NICE, put in the Appeal Hearings, 'we are held to account, quite properly, for what is said in it, and for the appropriateness and the quality, the relevance of the information on which the guidance is based' (Appeal Hearing Transcript: 130709: 97). This difference in the circles of accountability between NICE and clinicians was relevant in political terms and proved decisive in determining the development of the controversy.

Clinical Pragmatism and its Consequences

On the 10th of October 2006, NICE's Appeal Panel rejected the arguments put forward by the stakeholders. The Alliance re-affirmed its objections to the guidance. But something had changed. Immediately after appeals were rejected, the clinical bodies involved in the Alliance (RCP and British Geriatrics Society) issued a statement that aimed 'to support clinicians in preparing to meet their duties and responsibilities as doctors while implementing this flawed guidance' and recommended that 'clinicians should interpret the MMSE score in the light of the individual patient's circumstances' (Royal College of Psychiatry, 2006). The clinicians 'pragmatic' attitude to the guidance represented a withdrawal from direct confrontation with NICE but one that was underpinned by an insistence on clinical autonomy and the 'flawed' nature of NICE's guidance. This stemmed directly from the 'division of accountability' that NICE had proposed in the Appeal Hearings but also from their understanding of the MMSE as a rough, *malleable* tool (see above). It was as if clinicians were suggesting that clinical effectiveness could prevail despite the cost-effectiveness limits imposed on clinical practice.

This positioning was in a paradoxical relationship with the Alliance's public strategy and the public view of cost-effectiveness. Whereas before the Appeal Hearing public opinion was mostly supportive of the Alliance, after, a variety of actors voiced concern about the legitimacy of the Alliance's objections to NICE. Polly Toynbee, a left-leaning political commentator, writing in the Guardian, suggested that

> [a]ll kinds of agendas are at work in the attacks on NICE's decisions. The drug companies push for a yet fatter slice of NHS spending. Patient groups understandably want everything for their sufferers.[...] In the old days rationing was opaque, but now that it is transparent, can rational argument prevail with voters over rightwing tabloid agendas? [...] People know that there are always spending limits, and the NHS remains a great emblem of national solidarity (Toynbee, 2006).

Similar support for NICE was voiced in an Editorial in the *Lancet*,

> [NICE's decision] has been branded 'blatant cost cutting' by the Alzheimer's Society. But this reaction says less about NICE's decision-making processes— which are commendably rigorous—than about the gulf between patient expectations of the UK's tax-funded health system, and understanding about the necessity for rational spending (*Lancet*, 2006).

For lay and professional commentators, NICE's recommendation in relation to dementia drugs was underpinned by rationality and rigour. Cost-effectiveness judgements were necessary, particularly in a tax-funded health care system. If the NHS was to survive and pursue its value of solidarity, rationing was necessary. Opposition to NICE could only be motivated by 'agendas': the commercial interests of pharmaceutical companies, the expectations of patients and the political strategies of the media. Indeed, the fact that there was public opposition to NICE demonstrated that explicit rationing at work. For these commentators, cost-effectiveness had prevailed.

When, in January 2007, the Alzheimer's Society decided to join manufacturers in the application for a judicial review, this was no longer publicly seen as an articulation of 'reasonable concern'. Their defence of the clinical effectiveness of dementia drugs and their critique of cost-effectiveness was seen a divisive and sectional: the Alzheimer's Society was accused of playing into the strategies of the pharmaceutical industry and undermining the pursuit of reason, the NHS and its core values (Chalmers, 2007). The controversy had demonstrated that 'clinical effectiveness is insufficient for maintaining or introducing any clinical procedure' and that 'cost must also be taken into account' (Rawlins and Culyer, 2004).

Whither Clinical Effectiveness II?

In this chapter, I took as my point of departure the following question: how, when and for whom can cost-effectiveness be said to be more important than clinical effectiveness in the pursuit of health in contemporary societies? Contextualising the emergence of cost-effectiveness in an economic critique of clinical effectiveness, the chapter analysed how the establishment of systems of explicit rationing have sparked a variety of counter-critiques that emphasise the epistemic uncertainty of economic measurements of health and denounce their political assumptions and institutional supports (Crinson, 2004; Milewa, 2006). Focusing on the controversy over access to dementia drugs in the NHS, the chapter traced the construction, deconstruction and re-construction of an economic evaluation. It concluded that, in the case of dementia drugs, the stabilisation of a cost-effectiveness measurement – and of the use of cost-effectiveness evaluation in health care resource allocation – was underpinned by a 'division of accountability' where clinicians were to maintain their clinical autonomy in relation to the use of the MMSE as a 'rationing tool'. The securing of clinical autonomy allowed clinicians to re-affirm their epistemic commitment to a mechanical version of objectivity and their allegiance to clinical effectiveness.

This conclusion goes somewhat against sociological analyses of the relationship between assessments of clinical effectiveness and the maintenance of clinical autonomy. With the emergence of regulatory tools in medicine, sociologists and clinical bodies were quick to revisit the thesis that clinical autonomy was being eroded through processes of de-professionalisation and/or proletarianisation (Light and Levine, 1988). Timmermans and Berg proposed, drawing on Light's theory of countervailing powers (Light, 1991), that assessments of clinical effectiveness are part and parcel of a re-distribution of accountability within health care systems where third parties attempt to gain access to the 'black box' of clinical judgement (Timmermans and Berg, 2003). Whereas these analyses take the tension between clinical effectiveness and clinical autonomy as their conceptual anchor, if only to reconceptualise it, the case of the dementia drugs controversy demonstrates that they might be compatible in specific circumstances. The case study suggests that clinical effectiveness might be a resource through which clinicians defy further attempts to redistribute accountability within health care systems, particularly through the use of cost-effectiveness assessments. But the study also proposes that such defiance might be a resource for understanding the relationship between clinical and cost-effectiveness in contemporary health care systems. However, rather than seeing changes in this relationship as an effect of professional dynamics alone, the paper explored how demarcations within the controversy were linked to the mobilisation of divergent epistemic, institutional and political repertoires (Moreira, 2005).

These were related to three public conceptualisations of objectivity, of which only two became central for the resolution of the conflict. It could be argued that in the case presented here, clinicians' insistence on a mechanical interpretation of the MMSE was a response to NICE's unwillingness to accept the disciplinary, expertise-based version of objectivity (Porter, 1995: 4) that clinicians has proposed in 2001 and again in 2005–06. It was as if clinicians were suggesting that NICE was not playing according to their own rules. But in confronting NICE with its limitations, clinicians were doing more than being strategic. The analysis presented in the paper suggests that clinicians accepted that these were the terms of the engagement. Thus, I propose that the conflict between what I labelled 'regulatory' and 'mechanical' versions of objectivity is indicative of a wider shift in knowledge governance within health care. In this context, expert-based assessments are seen as insufficient to provide ground for public decision-making and rule-based, mechanical objectivity can no longer provide a suitable alternative. New forms of knowledge governance are needed but there is considerable uncertainty about when to deploy different models. Linked to a mechanical version of objectivity is the view that trials and other forms of health technology assessment should provide decision makers with accurate, robust evaluations of the impact of therapies on illnesses. Indicators of robustness such as validity or reliability dictate whether research should be used in practice and, in this, cost-effectiveness analyses should not be an exception. Regulatory objectivity emphasises the complex and heterogeneous character of knowledge-in-practice, where trials are but one of the possible sources of information. Knowledge robustness is still important but combined with reflexive explorations of the uncertainties and pragmatic links between research, practice and policy (Moreira, May and Bond, 2009). In the case presented here, the pragmatic reasoning went so far as to recognise how the standard might reasonably be ignored by practitioners. This is not an exception. Research on the use of cost-effectiveness analysis in health services (Light and Hughes, 2001; McDonald, 2002; Bryan et al., 2007; Williams et al., 2008) reveals that in actual allocative decisions economic models are but one of the dimensions decision makers take into consideration. From this perspective, the 'division of accountability' proposed by NICE should be seen as a token recognition of this complexity.

The same applies to the interpretation and use of clinical trial results. Within a regulatory objectivity framework, trials results become relevant to practice and policy through rich and contextualising analyses from a diversity of perspectives (see Will, this volume). This has consequences for how we might conceive of clinical effectiveness. Current models of evidence-based practice emphasise the interaction between research and clinical expertise (e.g. Sackett et al., 2000) and have been criticised for their 'mechanical' understanding of this relationship (Tanenbaum, 1994). This study suggests that there is an important, collective dimension to assessments of clinical effectiveness. In this, it is recognised that a variety of groups and forms of expertise have become integral to collective negotiations about what counts as clinical effectiveness. These processes explore and sometimes re-articulate the relationships between research, practice and policy within particular illness domains. They identify zones of uncertainty and ignorance, or mismatches between patients' needs and researcher's agendas.

However, while this approach is clearly embedded in actual collective decision making, official public discourse on the matter tends to emphasise the 'mechanical' aspects of evaluations of evidence. From this other perspective, NICE's proposed division of accountability served to reinforce the 'mechanical' version of clinical effectiveness. This in turn helped raise political support for explicit rationing in the NHS but only by obscuring the uncertainties and conventional aspects of the decision making process that had been explored during the controversy. If this analysis is correct, then it raises concerns about how public representations of the role of knowledge in health care might limit the knowledge generating capacities of collectives gathered around particular health issues and thwart the possibility of reinventing the meaning of clinical effectiveness.

PART III
Testing the Limits for Policy

In this third section, our contributors continue to probe questions about the effects of trials, looking in particular at their connections with the world of policy. It has frequently been suggested in the literature that trials may be used to support a technocratic approach to tricky questions of healthcare policy, especially prioritisation, at national and international levels. Thus trials may give authority to guidelines, which hold out the promise of standardised, costed approaches to prevention or treatment. The three final chapters consider the arguments made to support or reject the use of trials in public policy, investigating as they do the different 'publics' and 'patients' invoked in their organisation.

Dehue offers a historical discussion of the links between trials and policy, focussing less on the medical case than the application of the social sciences in other fields. If, as Faulkner suggests, the RCT appears to have become 'normal science' in healthcare, in Dehue's account this appears a rather late development in comparison with other areas of social policy, such as education, which experimented with aspects of trial methodology in the early 20th century. Dehue argues that experiences in these fields help reveal the assumptions behind trials, and thus their 'fit' with the needs of policy makers. This has three consequences: a focus on the individual as the location of both 'problem' and 'solution'; an interest in efficiency; and a tendency to reduce the space left for professional discretion. From debates about earlier social research, and political economy, she investigates opposition to these assumptions, and thus the applicability of these critiques to the current use of trials in healthcare. Her particular target is the almost exclusive focus on trials in recent Dutch guidelines on the treatment of depression. She argues that this reliance leads to an emphasis on pharmaceutical treatment for patients, whose illness is abstracted from the social and relational context of depression and efforts to mitigate it. In producing such 'abstract' patients, she suggests modern trials, and the policy they inform, continue to suffer from the decontextualisation that was identified by 19th century critics of the experimental method, and the 'artifical groups' created for comparison.

The other chapters in this section describe efforts to grapple more explicitly with issues of context, as the trial method is reinvented and reapplied to respond to the concerns of policy makers in very diverse settings. Both Kelly and Faulkner describe examples of what has been called 'effectiveness' research, linking these to a trend to 'socially robust knowledge' (Gibbons, 1999).

In Kelly's chapter the meaning of trials is negotiated against very different policy backgrounds in the UK and The Gambia. Trials in the UK build on existing infrastructure in a publicly funded health care system. In this situation, a 'pragmatic' trial of screening for osteoporosis can change practice as it incorporates it into the design of the trial, creating the conditions for the subsequent application of results across the country. In The Gambia, the context is more unstable and diversely populated, so that trial of screens to prevent mosquito-borne malaria becomes a temporary contract between specific communities and researchers funded by the UK's Medical Research Council (MRC). Though the relationship between the MRC and particular villages has developed over several decades, ultimately the MRC is quick to disinvest from these sites, leaving individuals to pay for malaria prevention and medical care in a situation where there is no government money for health services. The efforts of researchers to produce generalisable knowledge as a public good are therefore distressingly undermined by on the one hand the lack of a national policy audience, and on the other by the research community's sense of the project as ultimately too local.

Finally Faulkner offers a more optimistic account than either Dehue or Kelly of attempts by methodologists to develop clinical research that can account for and investigate the social relations that lie beyond trials. In particular he chronicles a set of extensions and adaptations to experimental methodology, which seek to explore and incorporate the beliefs and expectations of potential patients and take that knowledge into policy. The case is screening for prostate cancer: and he describes a situation in which the UK government is under pressure to decide how far to extend screening for the public, and in what form. Initially, the government appears to claim the 'need for research' as a way of buying time. Yet, as researchers debate trial design and start studies, the National Health Service becomes what he calls 'a distributed laboratory' for investigating the implications of screening. In particular, he notes that patient preferences are made the subject of new and careful investigation, as the state seeks to produce responsible and health-seeking citizens, as well as manage its costs.

Chapter 6

Comparing Artificial Groups: On the History and Assumptions of the Randomised Controlled Trial[1]

Trudy Dehue

In spring 2005, the 'Committee for Multidisciplinary Guidelines in Mental Health Care' in the Netherlands held a party. It celebrated the presentation of its 144 page *Multidisciplinary Guideline on Depression*, produced after several years of intense deliberations. The new guideline was meant to direct national decision-making in the treatment of clinical depression as well as administrative policies concerning mental health. The report of its 'festive presentation' described ambitious implementation plans such as a large-scale depression awareness campaign (Landelijke Stuurgroep multidisciplinaire richtlijnontwikkeling, 2005a). Yet, the joyous atmosphere at the party was a little forced. Not all members of the multidisciplinary group established in 1999 to produce the guideline were pleased with its result. As a matter of fact, the Netherlands Association of General Practitioners had refused to sign it, as had the Pandora Society, an organisation defending the interests of people with mental health problems.

These internal tensions in a medical guideline committee may not be unusual. The depression guideline in the Netherlands was primarily inspired by the ideal of evidence-based medicine (EBM) which proposes practice based on the results of randomised controlled trials (RCTs). After some more information about the implementation of these ideas in the Netherlands, I will embed this case in its historical and geographical context. My aim is to uncover some of the hidden assumptions in the RCT, assumptions which, as I will argue, are at the heart of disputes about the best treatment of depression in the Netherlands and elsewhere.

1   This chapter is partly a rewritten version of Dehue (2005) and Dehue (2008, chapter 6). I thank the publishing houses Wiley and Augustus for their permission to use these former publications: Dehue, T. (2005) History of the control group. In: *Encyclopedia of Statistics in the Behavioral Sciences, vol 2*. B. Everitt and D. Howell, eds. Copyright © 2005 John Wiley & Sons Ltd. (Reproduced with permission); and Dehue, T. (2008). *De Depressie-epidemie. Over de plicht het lot in eigen hand te nemen* [The Depression-epidemic. On the duty to manage one's destiny]. Copyright © Augustus. (Reproduced with permission.) I also thank Tiago Moreira, Ben Heaven and Catherine Will for their most helpful comments on a former version.

The 2005 Dutch guideline recommended antidepressants for cases of severe depression and either antidepressants or cognitive psychotherapy in less severe cases. In a letter written in December 2004, the Association of General Practitioners had communicated its view that with these recommendations the guideline 'cannot be laid down nor published.' The Association argued that the guideline group's preference for antidepressants was based on insufficient scientific grounds. Moreover, it maintained that it was not appropriate to restrict the word 'treatment' to therapies that could be tested in RCTs alone, arguing that in a family doctor's practice, advice and counselling are of major importance.[2]

In the same month, the Pandora Society had written a comparable letter, also protesting against the combination of reliance on experimental research and antidepressants. Trials testing medicines, the Society asserted, are often conducted in an improper way and even the outcomes of perfect trials cannot determine the best possible treatment for each individual patient. Moreover, the outcomes of RCTs may downplay the adverse effects and health risks of antidepressants as well as their detrimental effects on important aspects of daily life, which consumers regularly reported at the Pandora helpdesk. According to the Pandora Society the patients' own preferences and experiences should be taken much more seriously.[3]

These letters demonstrate that RCTs are not universally regarded as a gold standard, at least not in all contexts. Although the two protesting parties were in the minority in the Netherlands Task Group on Depression, their critique of the hegemony of experimentally acquired data is by no means unique. Ever since EBM has been equated with treatments positively tested in RCTs, opponents have called for a more personal approach in the practice of health care. They emphasise the need for careful searches for the right treatment for each individual rather than a standardised cure derived from average results obtained with groups of people.

The present chapter discusses similar arguments raised over a century ago. Most importantly, it investigates the implicit assumptions of the RCT by rewriting its standard history. Whereas many histories of the RCT aim to demonstrate that experimental group comparison has deep roots in the past of medical practice, this chapter considers the reasons that reputed 19th and early 20th century methodological experts like Adolphe Quetelet, John Stuart Mill and Frederick Stuart Chapin insisted for a long time that experimental group comparison was an unsuitable research method.

To be sure, the RCT is an indispensable research instrument. In addition, it has been impressively refined over the years. Yet, as I intend to show it is not the neutral research methodology many take it to be. Understanding the tacit assumptions of former scholars who rejected this method, helps to bring to light the tacit assumptions supporting the RCT in our own time. Simultaneously, such an analysis helps to explain why disputes about the RCT never died down completely.

---

2   The letter was published on http://nhg.artsennet.nl [accessed on 20 October 2007].

3   The letter was published on www.stichtingpandora.nl [accessed on 20 October 2007].

I begin with a section explaining how the standard historiography of the RCT renders its inherent assumptions invisible and then present an alternative history. At the end of the chapter, I return to the example of clinical depression in the early 21st century to draw out some of the implications of this historical analysis.

A Matter of Everyday Logic

There are many histories describing early cases of comparison between treated and untreated people. Most of them present these cases as a testimony to the long historical roots of the randomised controlled trial. For example, Jean Baptiste van Helmont, a Flemish doctor working in the 17th century, is often mentioned. He proposed studying the beneficial effects of leeches on human health by comparing people treated with those not treated with these blood-sucking creatures. Another famous example is that of James Lind's *A Treatise of the Scurvy*, published in 1783, which describes how Lind gave various treatments to sailors suffering from scurvy and carefully observed the results. The well-designed electronic library, www. jameslindlibrary.org, named after this 18th-century ship's doctor, provides many more examples. Although none of them fully meets the standards of contemporary RCTs, they are seen as precursors of the present.

Such histories describing founding fathers offer compelling stories. Professional historians, however, use a range of derogatory labels for them such as 'presentism,' 'finalism', 'feel good history', 'whig history' and 'preface history' (for example Kuhn, 1962). The reason is that such histories apply present-day standards in deciding which former authors should be included in the story and which fragments should be selected out of these authors' writings. Whereas these histories draw their own line from the present back into the past, they sketch a progressive trajectory from the past to the present. If contemporary views change, the preface-histories change along with them, highlighting other pioneers from the past with other practices. The present also serves to create coherence. The authors included may have lived miles or times apart and need not to have responded to one another's ideas, as the present standard serves as the 'glue' interconnecting the scattered fragments of the story. The effect is that the present acquires an aura of trans-historical, independent legitimacy.

Whereas this kind of history is rejected by professional historians for its historiographical flaws, one may also wonder whether checking the effects of an intervention through comparison with untouched cases is not a matter of simple everyday logic. Are examples of more or less standardised comparison in the history of medical practice really that special? Will builders, bakers and farmers not have done such checks as well? Indeed, further on in this chapter, agriculture will appear to have provided medicine with the statistical techniques for establishing the significance of differences between the results of the experimental and control groups.

Most importantly, given that examples of comparison in actual healing practices do indeed date back to ancient times, it is all the more remarkable that until the second half of the 20th century the most reputed methodological experts rejected it as a valid method for studying people. How to handle this discrepancy? Preface-histories typically do this by leaving former opponents of present-day beliefs out of the story, or by criticising them for the 'deficiencies' still present in their writings. This chapter, however, attempts to gain understanding of older methodological views that appear incongruous in the light of present standards. It does this by studying these views as contributions to debates in their own time. Likewise, it discusses the stances of later methodological experts who did advocate controlled trial methodologies in the context of debates with their own contemporaries. Only in this way can we understand how experimental comparison became a gold standard in methodological textbooks at a particular moment in time, first in psychology and somewhat later in medicine too. As I will argue, this shift required pivotal transitions in society at large, that is in assumptions about fair social relations as well as collective responsibilities, and in views of what it means to be an individual. This, of course, is not to deny the rationality of the RCT. It rather is to demonstrate that what may count as rational is unavoidably based on underlying culture-bound presuppositions. And it is to open up the possibility of discussions about the tenability of these presuppositions in various contexts, such as early 21st-century debates on the treatment of depression.

Incomparable Cases

Already in the 18th century, prominent scholars considered the value of experimentation as a method for investigating human life. In 1739, the Scottish philosopher David Hume, for instance, published a volume under the title of *Treatise of Human Nature. Being an Attempt to Introduce the Experimental Method of Reasoning into Moral Subjects*. As the title demonstrates, Hume used the expression of the 'experimental method' but he added the words 'of reasoning' since he was convinced that true experimentation with human beings was impossible. He and his Enlightenment contemporaries used the terminology of experimentation in a metaphorical sense for events happening anyway. Carefully observing the consequences of disturbances of regular life, they argued, was the human science substitute for experimentation in the natural sciences (Carrithers, 1995).

In the 19th century, scholars such as Adolphe Quetelet and John Stuart Mill, as well as Auguste Comte and George Cornewall Lewis, expressed similar views. They used the terminology of experimentation for incidents such as natural disasters, famines, economic crises, and administrative interventions into everyday life. True scientific experimentation with wilful manipulation by researchers, they too argued, was not feasible in the context of research with human beings. Hence, when the British mathematician and statesman Lewis published his two volume *Treatise on the Methods of Observation and Reasoning in Politics* (1852), he deliberately omitted the method of experimentation. Lewis argued that experimenting is 'inapplicable to man as a sentient, and also as an intellectual and moral being.' This is not, he added, 'because man lies beyond the reach of our powers' but because experiments 'could not be applied to him without destroying his life, or wounding his sensibility, or at least subjecting him to annoyance and restraint' (Lewis, 1852: 160–61).

Whereas these were ethical objections, there also were epistemological ones. Lewis' compatriot, the philosopher, economist, and methodologist John Stuart Mill considered experimentation with human beings impracticable. Mill's famous 1843 book *A System of Logic*, presented a range of research methods such as the 'method of difference' that entailed a systematic comparison of cases in which an effect does and does not occur. Although Mill regarded this as the 'most perfect of the methods of experimental inquiry', he argued that it was unsuitable in research with humans because in that case true comparability could not be achieved. He illustrated this with reference to the 'frequent topic of debate in the present century' on whether or not government intervention into free enterprise would impede national wealth. The method of difference was unhelpful in a case like this, he explained, because:

> [I]f the two nations differ in this portion of their institutions, it is from some differences in their position, and thence in their apparent interests, or in some portion or the other of their opinions, habits and tendencies; which opens a view of further differences without any assignable limit, capable of operating on their industrial prosperity, as well as on every other feature of their condition, in more ways than can be enumerated or imagined (Mill, 1843: 881–2).

Mill raised this objection of incomparability of cases not only in complex issues such as national economic policies but in relation to all research with people. Even the comparatively simple question of whether or not mercury cures a particular disease, was 'quite chimerical', he maintained, as it is impossible to isolate a single factor from all other ones that might constitute an effect. In medicine it was safer to rely on systematic observational research like in the examples of 'quinine, colchium, lime juice, and cod liver oil' that were shown to be beneficial in so many cases 'that their tendency to restore health [...] may be regarded as an experimental truth' (Mill, 1843: 451–2).

How could Lewis be scrupulous about individual integrity even to the level of fearing to 'annoy' people or 'wound their sensibility', when participation in an experiment could have been voluntary and be financially rewarded as it is today? And why did an astute methodologist like Mill not think of the solution, self-evident today, of simply composing comparable groups of patients if these do not exist in natural life? Briefly, how to explain the difference between these 19th-century methodological objections against experimentation and its broad acceptance among methodological experts in disciplines such as medicine and psychology in our own time?

European Urine

In 1865, the illustrious French physiologist Claude Bernard published a book with the deliberately provocative title of *Introduction à L'étude de la Médecine Expérimentale* translated into English as *Introduction to the Study of Experimental Medicine*. In contrast to his contemporaries, Bernard had no moral qualms about manipulation for the sake of research. 'Philosophic obstacles' to experimental medicine, he maintained, 'arise from vicious methods, bad mental habits and certain false ideas' and valid knowledge demands comparative experiments 'at the same time and on as comparable patients as possible' (Bernard, 1865: 194, 196).

Yet Bernard's experiments were only comparative in that sense that he often repeated his trials and looked for the most perfect one as the ideal case. One searches his *Introduction* in vain for experimental and control groups. This is because such experiments compare group averages whereas, as ardently as Bernard defended experimentation, he rejected the statistical mean. His *Introduction* fulminates page after page against the very idea. To illustrate its ludicrousness, Bernard for instance evoked the 'startling instance' of a colleague collecting urine 'from a railroad station urinal where people of all nations passed'. Anyone attaching value to the mean, he scoffed, apparently regards it useful to study 'l'urine *moyenne* Européenne!' ('the *average* European urine!'). Even mixing one person's urine produced in a day, would be nonsensical, he added, because that renders 'précisément l'analyse d'une urine qui n'existe pas' ('a perfect analysis of non-existing urine') (Bernard, 1865: 126).

Lewis's scruples, Mill's cautiousness, Bernard's grumpiness about the mean, all seem odd compared with modern conceptualisations of scientific research. From the perspective of the present-day gold standard these scholars were not yet fully aware of how proper research must be done (Brown, 1997a, 1997b). However, one can also ask whether or not ideas that look strange to us made sense in their own time. These 19th-century methodological notions become understandable in the framework of the organicist and determinist worldview of their time.

Organicism and Determinism

The word 'organicism' refers to the 19th-century conception of both communities and individuals as organic systems in which every element is closely related to all others. In such systems every characteristic is part of a unique pattern of interwoven strands rather than caused by one or more isolated variables acting in the same way in each case. Hence, not only countries but individuals too differed 'in more ways than can be enumerated or imagined', to repeat Mill's quote. And consequently, the urine of every living creature was part of its complete system that varies throughout the day, to use Bernard's example.

The word 'determinism' refers to the ascription of the facts of life to established laws of God or Nature rather than to human purposes and plans. According to 19th-century determinism, the possibilities of engineering human life were and should be limited. Rather than initiate permanent social change, the role of responsible authorities was to preserve public stability. Likewise, the assignment of responsible researchers was not to improve nature's design but to understand and preserve it. This point of view could lead to respect for nature and people but also to a kind of carelessness that seems unduly harsh nowadays. For instance, explaining that unfortunate events should be regarded as social experiments, Lewis easily combined his cautiousness about 'wounding' people's 'sensibility' with remarkable cold-heartedness about people's fate:

> A famine or a commercial crisis searches the weak points of a nation, and is sure to find them. It has an elective affinity with the rotten parts of the social fabric, and dissolves them by the combination. The study of monstrosities, or malformations, in the animal or vegetable kingdoms, has likewise been recommended as a means of tracing the laws of organic structure [...] Political institutions of an unusual and extraordinary character (which may be regarded as analogous to monstrosities in the organized world) may serve to throw light upon the corresponding institution in its ordinary form, and thus, to a certain extent, discharge the function of a scientific experiment (Lewis, 1852: 172–3).

Even Mill, to whom the injustice of *laissez-faire* economy was a significant topic, held that government interference should be limited to a small range of issues and should largely aim at the preservation of regular natural order (Kurer, 1991).

The same organicist and determinist philosophy expressed itself in 19th-century statistics where indeterminism was not yet something one should make good use of. Whereas today it sounds quite natural to derive the chance that a treatment will help a particular patient from earlier experiments, that did not make sense at the time. It was for this reason that Bernard not only sneered at physiologists 'mixing urine' but also at surgeons publishing the success rates of their operations. According to him, an average success did not give any certainty about the next operation to come and, hence, probabilistic statistics meant 'literally nothing scientifically' (Bernard, 1865: 137 and 195). Chance had the negative connotation of lack of knowledge and whimsicality rather than of something one should 'take' (Porter, 1986; Hacking, 1990).

For similar reasons, 19th-century statisticians doing population surveys did not take random samples but studied representative communities in their entirety (Porter, 1986; Desrosières, 1998). It would have been pointless to take individual people out of their natural habitat and compose a new artificial group lacking any social cohesion. To them that would have been like randomly taking ants out of various ant-nests and put them together in a new unnatural nest, which would make each ant a meaningless creature. And doing this in an effort to manipulate and improve the life of ants rather than merely understanding it.

It was because of their organicist (or holist) and determinist world view, that the idea of using chance for deriving population values or allocating individuals to artificial groups would have been senseless to these 19th-century scholars. Understanding the values that excluded the possibility of experimentation as a valid research strategy helps to recognise the 20th-century values legitimising it. The organicism and determinism of the 19th century had to make way for 20th-century elementarism and progressivism before comparing artificial groups could become a thinkable and valuable research tool.

The Profits of Piety

In the second half of the 19th century changes began to occur in both society and scientific methodology. The British statistician and biometrician Sir Francis Galton, for instance, did consider it his task to interfere in human life. He was intrigued by the evolutionary theory of his nephew Charles Darwin. However, whereas Darwin wanted to understand evolution, Galton aspired to enhance it. He also adopted and adapted the statistical mean for the sake of human progress.

The notion of the mean, rejected vehemently by Bernard, had been introduced by the Belgian mathematician Adolphe Quetelet who replaced the requirement of absolute laws stating that A is always B by that of statistical laws in which A can be B on average. In Quetelet's view that idea was in accordance with 19th-century determinism because to him the mean represented the ideal case. For example he measured the chest sizes of thousands of soldiers and regarded the average chest as a standard. Quetelet's famous *L'homme moyen* (average man) represented normalcy and dispersion from the mean signified abnormality. Unlike Bernard, Galton embraced Quetelet's average but he did reject Quetelet's interpretation of its meaning. He regarded Quetelet's equation of 'average' with 'normal' and 'ideal' as 'essentially unprogressive'. In an 1889 article, Galton argued about the average man that:

> [t]he class to which he belongs is bulky, and no doubt serves to keep the course of social life in action [...] But the average man is of no direct help towards evolution, which appears to our dim vision to be the primary purpose, so to speak, of all living existence [...] Some thoroughgoing democrats may look with complacency on a mob of mediocrities, but to most other persons they are the reverse of attractive (Galton, 1889: 406–7).

Galton already employed the mean in a progressive sense in an earlier article with the title 'Statistical Inquiries into the Efficacy of Prayer'. That article challenged religious people to study the beneficial effects of praying by investigating whether 'sick persons who pray, or are prayed for, recover more rapidly than others'.

Religious persons, Galton argued, might think that one can handle this question by simply studying a few 'isolated cases'. Against such a one-group approach he raised an objection that is fundamental to the later RCT. Anyone who only studies some isolated cases, he wrote, will 'run the risk of being suspected by others in choosing one-sided examples' (Galton, 1889: 126). Whereas Mill deemed the method of difference unfeasible in research with human beings and Bernard fiercely rejected the mean, Galton enthusiastically explained how sound experimental research of the profits of piety should be carried out:

> We must gather cases for statistical comparison, in which the same object is keenly pursued by two classes similar in their physical but opposite in their spiritual state; the one class being spiritual, the other materialistic. Prudent pious people must be compared with prudent materialistic people and not with the imprudent nor the vicious (Galton, 1889: 126).

As it seems, Galton was the first to advocate comparison of group averages in order to check whether a treatment has a beneficial effect. 'We simply look for the final result' he added optimistically, 'whether those who pray attain their objects more frequently than those who do not pray, but who live in all other respects under similar conditions'. Galton's prayer study, however, compared natural groups and was not yet an example of artificial groups created solely for the sake of research. In addition, it did not concern a treatment given solely for experimental purposes. For the emergence of this conception of experimentation, fears of being 'suspected by others in choosing one-sided examples' had to outgrow anxieties about disturbing organic wholes. This transition took place with the changeover from determinism to progressivism in society at large.

Three Maxims of Welfare Capitalism

Galton was not alone in his interest in progress. By the end of the 19th century, large numbers of agricultural workers had left their rural communities to become factory workers in the big anonymous cities of industrialised countries. The extreme destitution among them led to movements for the mitigation of *laissez faire* capitalism. Members of the upper middle class began to plead for state intervention via eugenicist programs, but also minimum wage bills, child labour bills, and unemployment insurance.

Appeals for an extension of government responsibility, however, also met with fears that governments would squander public funds and that help would reduce people's sense of their own responsibility. It was progressivism combined with such distrust that eventually constituted the definition of experimentation as statistical comparison of experimental and control groups. The process first took place in the United States. Three interrelated maxims of early 20th-century welfare capitalism were crucial to the gradual emergence of the present-day ideal.

The first maxim was that of individualism. That word has many meanings but here it refers to the elementarist notion that individual behaviour precedes society rather than the other way around. Individualism in this sense implies that people's health and success are predominantly the result of their own efforts and, consequently, that help should be limited. Ameliorative attempts had to be directed first and foremost at problematic individuals rather than structural change. Helping people implied educating, treating, punishing and rewarding them in order to turn them into independent citizens.

The second maxim was that of efficiency. Ameliorative actions financed with public money had to produce instant results with limited economical means. The fear that public funds would be squandered created a strong urge to attribute misery and backwardness to well-delineated causes rather than complex patterns of social relations.

The third maxim was that of impersonal procedures. Fears about possible abuse of social services evoked distrust in their own claims about their needs and the search for impersonal techniques to establish the truth behind their stories. It was not only that the self-assessment of potential recipients was to be distrusted, but the interests of the people providing help also gave cause for concern. Measurement also had to limit the discretion of professionals and to control their claims of efficiency (Porter, 1995).

Academic experts on political, economical, psychological, and sociological issues adapted their former philosophical questions and theoretical approaches to the new demands. They began to produce technically useful data collected according to standardised methodological rules. Moreover, they established a partnership with statisticians who now began to focus on population variability rather than communality in an attempt to establish the causes of the problems that had to be solved. In this context, the traditional interpretation of chance as mere whimsicality was replaced by chance as something to make good use of. As in Galton's writings, the statistical mean gained a positive reputation as an indication of the chance that a remedy is effective (Porter, 1986; Hacking, 1990; Desrosières, 1998).

The new social scientists measured people's abilities, motives, and attitudes, as well as social phenomena such as crime, alcoholism, and illiteracy. Soon, they arrived at the idea that their tests might as well be used for establishing the results of ameliorative interventions. In 1917, the American sociologist Frederick Stuart Chapin discussed this issue at length. Simple before and after measurement of one group, he stated, would not suffice to exclude personal judgement from the evaluation of interventions. Yet Chapin still rejected comparison of treated and untreated groups. Using a 20th-century version of Lewis' 19th-century moral objections, he argued that it would be immoral to withhold help from needy people just for the sake of research. And like Mill before him, he maintained that fundamental differences between groups would always invalidate the conclusions of the experiments (Chapin, 1917a; 1917b).

Matching Children

Unlike sociologists, psychologists in this period could draw on a tradition of experimentation. In 19th-century laboratory research they had studied the law-like relationships between physical stimuli and mental sensations with small groups of volunteers. During the combined administrative turn of government and human science, many of these psychologists too adapted their psycho-physiological research methods to the new demands of establishing progress rather than natural laws. They mostly offered their services for the enhancement of efficiency in education, which was a veritable movement in the United States (Danziger, 1990).

Just like the volunteers in the earlier psycho-physiological experiments, schoolchildren and their teachers were easily persuaded to cooperate in psychological experiments. Whereas sociologists like Chapin deemed it impossible to find comparable groups, creating artificial groups that exist only for the sake and the duration of an experiment appeared unproblematic in the school setting. Psychological experimenters tested the educational effects of fresh versus ventilated air, memorising methods, and pedgogical measures such as punishing or praising by comparing groups composed for the sake of research. During the 1920s, it became customary to handle the problem of possible differences between natural groups by the method of 'matching'. For instance, in order to find out whether or not praise makes a difference to educational outcomes, it was held that the groups should not differ in intelligence. Hence, pairs of children were created by selecting those with similar results on an intelligence test, then assigning one to the praise (experimental) group and the other to the no-praise (control) group.

The matching procedure, however, needed to be repeated for every thinkable factor that might create bias. Maybe the social background of the children would also make a difference, or their religion? Hence, matching was time consuming and expensive. In addition, it depended on the imaginative power as well as reliability of the researchers involved. This technique only accommodated possible confounding factors of which the designers of an experiment were aware, for which they were able to pre-test the participants, and which they did not disregard out of wishful thinking. In sum, although the new procedure obeyed the principle of individualism, it violated those of efficiency and impersonality.

These problems were solved in the early 1920s by assigning the children to the groups on the basis of chance. A 1923 methodological manual *How to Experiment in Education* argued that enhancing the efficiency of education could save billions of dollars and also proposed to use random allocation to the groups as 'an economical substitute' for matching (McCall, 1923: 41–2).

The Expansion of the RCT

Gradually the idea of comparing randomly composed groups spread among other educational psychologists. In addition, researchers began to test more than one variable simultaneously which made the data hard to handle. The methodological handbook *The Design of Experiments*, published in 1935 by the British biometrician and agricultural statistician Ronald Fisher, provided the solution of 'analysis of variance' (ANOVA). When working as a visiting professor at the agricultural station of Iowa State College in the United States, Fisher met the American statistician George Snedecor. In 1937, Snedecor published a book based on Fisher's statistical methods that was easier to comprehend than Fisher's own writings and was widely read by methodologists in psychology. In 1940, the educational psychologist Everett Lindquist, followed with the book *Statistical Analysis in Educational Research* that became a much-cited source in the international educational community (Lovie, 1979; Rucci and Tweney, 1980).

To Fisher random allocation was primarily a statistical condition for the validity of his ANOVA technique. Yet, his help was also welcomed with open arms by administrators because it helped to ensure the maxim of impersonal procedures from the very start of an experiment. As Snedecor expressed it in 1936: '[n]o more than a decade past, the statistician was distinctly on the defense' but '[u]nder the leadership of R.A. Fisher, the statistician has become the aggressor' (Snedecor, 1936: 690). Stated differently, statisticians too began to regulate the conduct of researchers. The desire to remove discretion, and reduce costs, drove the move to substitute matching by randomisation. Like Galton in 1872 who warned against eliciting accusations of having chosen one-sided examples, early 20th-century statisticians and methodologists cautioned against the danger of selection bias caused by high hopes of particular outcomes.

To 19th-century scholars like Lewis experimentation was 'inapplicable to man as a sentient, and also as an intellectual and moral being.' However, as 19th-century *laissez-faire* capitalism was replaced by 20th-century welfare capitalism, it became more acceptable to interfere in people's lives for the sake of progress and hence to allocate them to experimental and control groups. In the United States in particular, numerous RCTs have been done to test administrative interventions. The typical subjects were students, soldiers, patients, criminal offenders, drug abusers, incompetent parents, spouse beaters, and people on welfare who are comparatively compliant with an experimental regime (Boruch, 1997; Orr, 1999). In psychology and sociology this type of experimentation became the standard to such an extent that the expression 'randomised controlled trial' did not become current in these disciplines. Just 'the' experiment suffices because other kinds of methods became 'quasi-experiments' at best (Cook and Campbell, 1979).

For generations, students in the social sciences have learned that 'the experiment' is a neutral research instrument. Yet, its design still epitomises the maxims of individualism, efficiency, and impersonality that were embedded in its early development. As the comparison with 19th-century organicism clarifies, taking individuals out of their normal context and studying them in newly created artificial groups can only make sense if we assume that the problem to be solved is not a contextual one and is fully located in the individual. Something similar holds true for the maxim of efficiency embodied in the RCT. Tracing singular variables and comparing averages on these variables only makes sense if one supposes that singular variables are relevant and that one particular treatment will be best for everybody. Finally, the core of the RCT is that it bans personal discretion and relies instead on impersonal procedures. That is a wise thing to do, provided that the interpretations of the people being studied and treated are indeed insignificant, along with those of their doctors, therapists, teachers, family or friends.

Regulating Doctors and Manufacturers

In medicine too the demands of individualism, efficiency and impersonal procedures became increasingly important across the 20th century. For instance, in the course of time, the image of disease became elementaristic. Whereas formerly every individual's disease resulted from a unique pattern of factors such as the person's constitution, behaviour, and general conditions of life, by the end of the 19th century diseases became entities in themselves striking everyone in a similar way. This transition from, what medical historians call 'a holistic to an entity model of disease' (Rosenberg, 2002; 2003) was necessary for the RCT to become a useful instrument in medicine because in a holistic medical world it makes no sense to allocate people randomly to groups or to derive the best treatment for an individual from group averages.

Whereas educational administrators had to control school managers and teachers, medical administrators had to regulate the much more powerful pharmaceutical companies and self-assured medical professionals. An extensive system of regulations was established in order to enforce collaboration by industry. In addition, many thousands of doctors had to be regulated who were used to their status of an elite deciding at its own discretion. For the multifaceted and laborious history of this process, I refer to other historians (FDA, 1981; Marks, 1997; Daemmrich, 2004).

Nevertheless, in the context of the present history it is important to note that many medical practitioners expressed qualms that justified distrust of pharmaceutical companies began to determine the relationship between doctors and patients as well. Whereas they too regarded it dangerous to rely on pharmaceutical companies' own judgment when it comes to licensing newly designed medicines, these physicians maintained that in a doctor's office seasoned discretion is indispensable. If EBM was to be solely based on RCTs, the doctor had to become a technician acting according to pre-established rules rather than a personal advisor. In actual practice, many doctors countered in a holist way, the best treatment for an individual also depends on his or her other complaints, history, social circumstances, own preferences, habits, and beliefs. In addition, the hope and trust that RCTs are supposed to eliminate, are important healing factors in clinical settings.

Understandably, the advocates of experimentation in medicine, like those in educational research, welcomed the statistician as 'the aggressor', to repeat Snedecor's quote. In medicine too, it was Fisher's work, with his requirement of random allocation for the sake of sound analysis of variance, that helped to enforce objectivity defined as impersonal judgment (Marks, 1997).[4] The British epidemiologist Austin Bradford Hill is known as the first one to apply Fisher's technique in medicine while testing streptomycin for pulmonary tuberculosis in the 1940s. The earliest examples of randomised controlled trials with psychopharmaceuticals such a chlorpromazine and lithium followed in the 1950s (Marks, 1997; Healy, 1997).

In the course of time, objections against the RCT began to sound like mere excuses of an older generation unwilling to give up its elitist position. In many countries, regulating authorities and insurance companies now demand that the efficacy or effectiveness of all kinds of treatments has been demonstrated with randomised controlled trials. When the expression 'evidence based medicine' made its entry in the 1990s, it rapidly became synonymous with medicine based on results of RCTs. Yet, protests about this equation have not fully died down as the example of resistance against the 21st century Netherlands' *Multidisciplinary Guideline on Depression* demonstrates.

What Counts as Evidence?

Academic communities in social science, psychology and medical science in the Netherlands are inspired mostly by Anglo-Saxon research traditions. In this country too the RCT is generally considered the best instrument for establishing the efficacy of treatments for the reasons described in the previous sections. Consequently, the majority of members of the task group that was responsible for the depression guideline in the Netherlands maintained that the results of RCTs should direct its decisions. Yet, the status allocated to antidepressants in the guideline was higher than the Association of General Practitioners and the Pandora Society would have wished. In their eyes, not only do the necessarily short RCTs underestimate the adverse effects of medicines, in cases of depression personal preferences and individual approaches are of major importance. The

---

4   The importance of Fisher's statistical theory for the use of random allocation in the streptomycin trial is a complex issue. Though the vocabulary reflects Fisher's work, in that particular instance Bradford Hill may have been more concerned with 'clinical' than 'statistical' issues, in seeking to conceal allocation from physicians and patients, managing the risk of investigator bias (see Chalmers, 2005) continuing the trend to use methodological innovation to produce 'impersonal judgement' described above – Editors.

previous sections demonstrated that both protesting parties have important allies in the past, but they also have them in the present.

Many contemporary adherents of psychodynamic therapies, for instance, feel that the basic principles of their approach are violated when tested with an RCT. They contrast the model of depression as an entity striking everyone in a similar way to a model of depression as a response to events in someone's personal life. Consequently, in their view the diagnosis and the treatment of depression should not focus on isolated variables nor be derived from average efficacy in other people. Instead, a person's individual history should be understood and carefully analyzed. The personal relation between therapist and client is of pivotal importance as are the patients' own beliefs and preferences. In addition, the definition of efficacy in psychodynamic therapies is different from that in randomised clinical trials. Rather than measure patients' progress on a number of test items, a psychodynamic treatment aims at helping a patient to gain self-knowledge and to live with his or her losses and limitations (Jarvis, 2004). Stated in historical terms, psychodynamic therapies are based more on 'holist and determinist' than on 'elementarist and progressive' assumptions. The principles of individualism, efficiency and impersonal procedures that brought about the RCT help to explain why psychodynamic therapists – just like the general practitioners in the Netherlands – have often argued that RCTs disregard the essence of their work (Jarvis, 2004; Leichsenring, 2005).

Historical and sociological explanations of human fears and despair that point at factors like the increase of social inequality in advanced western societies are also based on 'holistic' rather than elementaristic assumptions (Bauman, 2007; Friedli, 2009; Wilkinson and Pickett, 2009). They study people as part of communities shaped by historical developments rather than as separate individuals. As John Stuart Mill argued, it is impossible to experiment with communities as they differ 'in more ways than can be enumerated or imagined.' Hence, in countries like the Netherlands where the RCT became the gold standard, such sociological, historical and theoretical research has less scientific status because it can be correlational or analytical 'at best.' In this situation the societal factors causing unhappiness tend to disappear from sight.

Most importantly, the RCT also has its limitations in medicine. Certainly it would be dangerous to clear the path for ineffective and unsafe drugs or to rely on 'eminence based' rather than evidence based drug treatments. Yet, it may also be dangerous to rely solely on the RCT. An additional cause for concern here is the commercialisation of clinical trial research, which I will not discuss in the present chapter.[5] Apart from the urgent need for independently financed trials, however, there is also a need to acknowledge the inherent limitations of the RCT. The ideal

---

5   This aspect is extensively discussed in Dehue (2008), chapter 7 and 8. Some of the manifold recent publications about it in English are Angell, 2004; Turner, E.H., et al., 2008, Sismondo, 2008; Garratini and Chalmers, 2009; PloS Medicine editors, 2009.

of strict and standardised comparison has its advantages but also creates its own problems.

To begin with, it is important to note that those relying on RCTs tend to regard improvement due to attention as a 'mere' placebo-effect which suggests that only medicines can be veritable treatments.[6] Furthermore, an effect during an experiment does not guarantee an effect in real life. People in artificial groups studied in artificial settings may react differently in daily life where problems are more multi-faceted and where one is not constantly monitored. The standardised diagnostic tests used in experimental research also demand that participants express their emotions in pre-established formats and reduce their personal stories to grades on a depression-scale (Healy, 2009; Dehue, 2002; Helms, 2002; Rapley et al., 2006).

Just like Bernard in the 19th century, present-day critics also argue that an effect of a drug on a particular individual cannot be predicted with certainty from average experimental results obtained with trial participants. People differ and what is beneficial to some is not necessarily beneficial to everyone. Present-day pharmacogenetic research appears to support Bernard's position by pointing out that genetic variation may be the cause of lack of efficacy in many people. In clinical trials, such inter-individual differences may be averaged out. The same holds for the discovery of side-effects. Many argue that much more serious monitoring of consumers is necessary after a drug has been licensed, as pre-licensing trials are not able to identify important safety problems with drugs used in everyday practice. For instance, in 2002 the WHO issued a strong warning about the magnitude of this issue, arguing that 'the patients used in clinical trials are selected and limited in number, the conditions of use differ from those in clinical practice and the duration of the trials is limited' (WHO, 2002: 8). The example of repeated reports of severe aggression and suicides after the consumption of SSRI's in particular indicates that regulators have relied too much on clinical trials alone (Medawar et al., 2003; Boyer and Shannon, 2005).

As Annemarie Mol has cogently argued treating diabetes patients simply at the basis of the outcomes of RCTs would be a matter of neglect, because these patients not unlike people suffering from depression, each have their own personal story and circumstances (Mol, 2008). Careful monitoring of each unique patient who starts using medication remains necessary, even if the treatment is based on convincing RCTs. In Germany the results of RCTs have acquired less authority than in the US (Daemmrich, 2004). Consequently, German doctors keep a better eye on patients who take medicines by questioning and examining them. They also report adverse events more actively to databanks and have developed better statistical methods in Germany to analyze such data (Daemmrich, 2004).[7]

---

6   A more positive name for the 'placebo effect' is the 'meaning response' (Moerman, 2002).

7   Some more recent publications warning against too much reliance upon RCTs are Kaptchuck, 2001; Parker, Anderson and Haddad, 2003; Healy, 2009; McGoey, 2010. Special

Coda: Struggling with Depression in the Netherlands

This chapter ends with some of the more recent history of depression treatments in the Netherlands. In response to the events described above, the Association of General Practitioners decided to write its own guideline whereas the Pandora Society kept on staffing its telephone helpline as well as issuing warnings about side-effects of antidepressants (until, in February 2010, it had to stop its activities when the government withdrew its funding after 40 years).

Meanwhile, the Netherlands Health Council based its national protocol for depressed employees on the contested multidisciplinary guideline and hence also advances antidepressants as the first treatment of choice (Gezondheidsraad, 2006). The health insurers in the country did the same, adding that psychotherapeutic treatments should be as brief as possible whereas the consumption of antidepressants should be continued for 6 months after recovery (Zorgverzekeraars Nederland and GGZ Nederland, 2008).

However, since this guideline was issued, international debates about antidepressants have continued with an increasing number of publications severely doubting the efficacy and safety of these medications (Kirsch et al., 2008; Turner et al., 2008; Ioannidis, 2008; Fournier et al., 2010). Whereas the reported effects of antidepressants in the 2005 guideline already were rather limited with only 20% of the participants in published RCTs showing more progress on a real antidepressant than on a placebo,[8] a subsequent depression guideline committee installed in 2007 and working in 2008 to revise the guideline had a number of such new trials at its disposal.

This committee's new draft guideline was made public on the internet in February 2010. It repeats the principle that the RCT is the gold standard of research. However, it also argues that cognitive and behavioural therapies have been shown to be as effective as antidepressants. Antidepressants should be preserved for 'therapy-resistant' and severe long-lasting depression, according to this guideline (Consortium Richtlijnontwikkeling, 2009; Bockting, Boerema and Hermens, 2010). The Association of General Practitioners accepted the new guideline. When the present chapter went to the press it was too early to make any predictions about its further reception.

---

journal issues critically discussing the RCT are; *Perspectives in Biology & Medicine* (2005, 48, 4) and *Biosocieties* (2007, 2, 2).

8   The guideline stated that 50–55% of the participants in RCTs improve for 50% or more, but also added that 30–35% in the placebo groups do too (Landelijke Stuurgroep multidisciplinaire richtlijnontwikkeling, 2005b, pp. 56–9).

Chapter 7

Pragmatic Fact-making: Contracts and Contexts in the UK and the Gambia

Ann Kelly

> The commitment with MRC [UK Medical Research Council] *is on contract*. But though we have the interest and the willingness to participate with MRC, let us pray that there will be a *continual extension of this contract*.
>
> (Alkalo of Pallen Fulla, The Gambia 02.20.2005, emphasis added)

This chapter is intended to cut across certain ways of thinking about *the context* of research as an element of its empirical content and ethical practice. It follows a provocation by Nowotny, Gibbons and Scott in their analysis of contemporary knowledge production, which describes the increasing role of society in science as a process of contextualisation (1994; 2001). The suggestion is that in a political era in which technological innovation provides both the benchmark for social progress and the infrastructure for economic development, the value of research is vetted within specific policy environments. At the same time, the ever tighter interlocking of science and capital has blurred the demarcations of public, state and commercial institutions; industries have been denationalised, privatisation policies have moved governmental and academic institutions into the market place.[1] Under these conditions, Nowotny, Gibbons and Scott argue, the value of science is no longer the prerogative of impartial expertise. Rather, it is the product of a dynamic collaboration among researchers, government, industry, and an informed public (e.g. Irwin and Wynne 1996; Nowotny et al., 2002; Jasanoff, 2005). This epistemic register, defined by an embrace of the context in which research takes place, indicates 'a shift from the search for "truth" to the more pragmatic aim of providing a provisional understanding of the empirical world that "works"' (Gibbons, 1999: 3). In their view, empirical pragmatics provides the ground for a new social contract posed between researchers, government and its citizens. Significantly,

---

1   In *The New Production of Knowledge* (1994), Nowotny, Scott, and Gibbons describe this transformation as a shift from a form of knowledge production that is objective, disinterested (what they term Mode 1) to one that is comprehensive, socially embedded and capable of reflexive management (Mode 2). In their sequel, *Rethinking Science* (2001), the authors explore the emergence of Mode 2 knowledge production as it relates to wider social transformations – the co-evolution of science and society.

as its purpose is no longer to sustain the production of disinterested knowledge, the terms of the new social contract depart from a bureaucratic model, whereby society speaks through its representative institutions.[2] Abandoning the notion that left to its own devices, science will produce public good, this new social contract comes about through lay participation and interdisciplinary experimentation; it is an 'embedded process in which all the contingencies, constraints and opportunities created by contextualisation would be made more explicitly and therefore capable of reflexive management' (Nowotny et al. 2001: 65).[3]

The participatory quality of this avowedly new contract raises immediate questions of method. Though policy may adopt a language of public-engagement, scholars have raised questions as to how, exactly, social value is internalised through scientific *practice*, and in what ways society is or can be taken into account (e.g. Barry 2001; Hayden, 2003; Miller, 2005; Strathern, 2002)? This chapter takes up this methodological query by looking at two public health experiments: the first investigates the effectiveness of a clinical screening program for osteoporosis in the UK; the second examines the effectiveness of household screening for the prevention of malaria in the Gambia. Pragmatic in approach, both trials are, in markedly different ways, exemplars of contextualised knowledge. They were designed to pilot policy and to offer a *realistic* gauge of public health impact. The experimental context generated by these trials sought to account for the unpredictability associated with routine delivery.[4] Significantly, they also both work to transform the context in which they take place, by reorganising the healthcare practices of their participant populations.

To the extent to which these trials provide empirical traction to the relationship between science and society, the argument of this chapter follows the path laid out by Nowotny, Gibbons and Scott. In their account, clinical research exemplifies the epistemic and ethical value of contextualisation (2001: 40, 132, 148–50, 211). The chapters in this volume indicate why this might well be the case. Medical research is a practice that crosses several intellectual and institutional domains. The methodological precision of clinical research does not ensure its epistemic value; the risks incurred by the subject demand that clinical trial outcomes benefit the population at large. Medical hypotheses are probed in the clinic and shaped to

---

2   As Gibbons puts it: 'under the prevailing contract between science and society, science has been expected to produce "reliable" knowledge, provided merely that it communicates its discoveries to society. A new contract must now ensure that scientific knowledge is "socially robust", and that its production is seen by society to be both transparent and participative' (Gibbons, 1999: 81).

3   For beyond a preoccupation with utility, Nowotony, Gibbons and Scott identify the pragmatic dimensions of this new science as the integration of ethical, legal and financial considerations into the assessment of research aims and outcomes.

4   The methodological literature describes this distinction as one between 'efficacy' and 'effectiveness'. The pragmatic method is first mentioned 1967 (Schwartz and Lellouch 1967: 637–48).

address the priorities of health policy. Thus the value of clinical research cannot be disentangled from the context in which it takes place: its scope is delimited by the *relevance* of its claims. But unlike other modes of research, because publics are already physically included in the research as participants, the issue of how to reflexively manage experimentation gains considerable amplitude (Strathern, 2000). The alignments that clinical research must generate between actors, resources, objects, knowledges and practices provide a model investigative format for the kind of complex collaboration that Nowotny, Gibbons and Scott believe the new social contract demands (Hayden, 2007).

In drawing material from research conducted in the developing world, this chapter seeks to complicate this line of reasoning. In Africa, as in Europe, public engagement in science has become a central issue for research policy and practice. Here too, scholarship underscores the need to integrate contextual concerns into the design and conduct of clinical trials: 'public consultation forums', 'community partnerships', and 'stakeholder meetings' are now a standard feature of transnational research enterprise (Binka, 2005; Benatar, Singer and Daar, 2005; Leach, Scoones and Wynne, 2005; Nuffield Council on Bioethics, 2005; WHO, 2006). However, despite the comparable framing of the social value of science as a process of taking society into account, for transnational medical research, contextualisation emerges as an issue of ethics. Situations of health and economic crisis, for instance, introduce implicit forms of coercion into subject enrolment, placing barriers to the possibility of genuine consent and to the generation of lasting benefits (Angell, 1997; Molyneux and Geissler, 2008). Community-engagement strategies aim to minimise the potential for exploitation by expanding the remit of research to consider 'the best interests of whole populations … and the ethics of international relations' (Benatar and Fleisher, 2007: 618). That process of taking society into account is pitched towards the expectations of healthcare that arise during research and not towards transforming the objects and practices of science itself. In short, an ethical approach to contextualisation consists *in adding provisions on to research* to compensate for the infrastructural gaps between research, health policy and practice.

This chapter bridges and develops these two discussions about the social value of research in Europe and in the developing world. In so doing, I hope to add ethnographic texture to the concept of a contract between science and society and, hopefully, gain a greater appreciation of the possibilities and limitations of contextualisation in advancing that relationship. Foregrounding the 'pragmatic' character of these projects, I want to consider how the context is incorporated into practice, and the social and scientific mileage that accommodation entails. The juxtaposition of these two cases arguably produces some predictable conclusions. In the UK, the context of research describes an institutional location; the social and material links generated through the processes of research serve to transform diagnostic practice for osteoporosis in the NHS. In the Gambia, the pragmatic tactics to remake domestic space as protective against malaria do not scale-up – they remain attached to the architecture of experimental household. Here, the context describes an *ethical technique* – an effort to respond to participant demands enrolled in a specific experiment (Franklin, 2003). However, instead of reducing this difference to the intractable nature of research conducted without the appropriate infrastructure, I argue that the way the social is conceptualised – epistemologically or ethically – has considerable consequences for the form of the public good these trials can generate (Strathern, 2002).

SCOOP (SCreening Of Older women for Prevention of fractures)

Because medical research strives to be representative of the realities of health care, the boundary that separates a clinical experiment from the external world is more porous than the characteristic lab sciences (Latour and Woolgar, 1979). However, the degree to which external contingencies should be incorporated into clinical trial design, the relative benefits and potential biases of standardised settings have polarised debate for decades. The evidence-based medicine (EBM) movement has sought to realign clinical authority with the evidentiary standards of biomedicine, linked to the randomised controlled trial (RCT).[5] However, for professionals concerned with the quality of health care delivery – and not simply the efficacy of an intervention under ideal conditions – the highly controlled-setting of the RCT may appear unrepresentative of the realities of health care, and thus fails to meet the practical needs of clinical decision makers (Timmermans and Angell, 2001; Maesneer et al. 2003). The reliability of research-generated data depends more on the utility of its findings than on the stability of its controls (Godwin et al. 2003; Tunis, Stryer and Clancy, 2003; Will, 2007).[6] In recent years, clinical researchers have begun to develop hybrid research designs to generate practical information to guide routine practice rather than explanatory data about the pharmacological or physical effects of an intervention (e.g. Kachur et al., 2001; Macpherson, 2004). This approach strives to balance methodological rigour with clinical relevance, by taking into account the vicissitudes of physician care and patient health (Wood, Ferlie, and Fitzgerald, 1998; Grol and Grimsaw, 2003).

My understanding of the methodological challenges attendant to clinical research is drawn from fieldwork conducted with the Arthritis Research Campaign (ARC), a UK-based charity that sponsors clinical trials in rheumatology. During the January 2004 funding meeting of the ARC Clinical Trials Collaboration (CTC), an application to conduct a 'pragmatic randomised controlled trial of the effectiveness and cost effectiveness of screening for osteoporosis in older women

---

5   Sackett's frequently-cited definition of EBM reflects these concerns by encompassing both the science and the art of medicine, the production of knowledge and its application (Sackett et al., 1996, 71).

6   The empirical trade-off is often phrased in terms of sacrificing 'internal coherence' for 'external validity'; while large-scale RCTs with clear-cut endpoints often produce elegant results, pragmatic evidence is believed to be more clinically relevant.

in the prevention of fractures' attracted the committee's attention. The application earned high marks from external reviewers for 'the significance of its question' and was selected by the committee as a particularly strong candidate for ARC support. Though some concerns were raised about the trial's design, the ARC agreed to finance the trial as an eighteen-month feasibility study involving 800 female patients over the age of 70 at two Primary Care Trusts.[7] Now expanded into a seven-year project (2007–2014), the SCOOP (SCreening Of Older women for Prevention of fractures) Trial has recruited 11,600 women aged between 70 and 85 across seven sites in the UK.[8]

The trial investigates a screening program that combines clinical examination with a DEXA scan, an x-ray technology that determines a patient's bone mineral density. Though there is little doubt that the DEXA scan is the gold standard for diagnostic practice (Ferguson, 2004: 180), what concerns the SCOOP's principal investigator is that 'treatment for osteoporosis is expensive and scanning machines are not readily available.'[9] The trial, therefore, is directed toward the problem of distribution: for what group of people, at what time in their lives, will the assessment of fracture risk by DEXA be most beneficial and least costly to the National Health Service (NHS)?[10] To answer this question requires, first, an intervention that combines technological and clinical elements. To that end, the research team plans to incorporate the scan within a program that effectively links patient self-assessment with General Practitioner (GP) diagnosis. Addressing the impact of such a program on both patient and institutional outcomes necessitates a proof that will demonstrate those complex and context-specific therapeutic relations (Campbell et al., 2000).[11]

---

7   Primary Care Trusts are statutory bodies responsible for delivery of health care and the provision of community health services to a local area. Within the parameters of the budgets and priorities set by the Strategic Health Care Authority, they can fund GPs and commission hospital services from NHS trusts or the private sector.

8   In January 2005, the ARC CTC awarded £200,000 to conduct a twelve-month pilot study across two Primary Care Trusts in Norwich and Sheffield. In 2006, this amount was increased to £380,000, and with the combined support of the Osteoporosis Society the SCOOP trial has begun enrolment (for more information see http://medtrials.uea.ac.uk/scooptrial).

9   Personal communication, Lee Shepstone, 12th November 2005.

10   This information is drawn from a series of interviews and conversations conducted by the author with the PI, Dr Lee Shepstone (2004–2005), and from the initial grant application for the trial (Shepstone, Harvey and Fordham 2004).

11   To determine the effectiveness of this intervention, the team had to take into account the number of osteoporotic patients identified, the subsequent effectiveness of the treatment, the cost of the program measured in time, money, and potential side-effects, and the ease with which GPs might integrate the technique into practice. The expertise necessary for this research required the formation of a multidisciplinary research team comprising orthopaedic specialists, rheumatologists, public health specialists, economists, and statisticians.

On the broadest level, the purpose of the trial will be to demonstrate how an osteoporosis-screening program might work in 'everyday practice'. That challenge is primarily one of design: how can a trial simultaneously model a clinical interaction and measure its effects on patient and clinician behaviour? The research team addressed this problem by deploying an intriguing protocol. At the start of the trial, the GP sends a letter to female patients aged seventy to eighty-five asking them if they would like to participate in a study. The letter is accompanied by a consent form, information leaflets on osteoporosis, and a baseline information booklet designed to assess a patient's overall risk of fracture. Those patients who agree to participate are randomised into a control and a screening group. From clinical information provided on participant self-assessment forms, the GPs then divide the screening group into three subsets. The first group, considered to be at low risk, will not be contacted further.[12] The second group, found to be at high risk, will be given appointments to discuss disease management. The third group, whose level of risk could not be assessed from the self-reported forms, will have their bone mineral densities measured by a DEXA scanner. If the scanning determines that a patient is at high risk for a fracture, a course of treatment will be recommended.

When it was initially presented, the trial raised a number of methodological problems for the ARC funding committee. With regards to the patient volunteers, would the use of self-assessment forms and the distribution of informational leaflets generate an unusually proactive sample population? Might the information provided about osteoporosis alter the conduct of the control group? Now more aware of the risks associated with the disease, would not all those enrolled in the trial be more likely both to seek treatment and to adopt behaviours that would reduce their risk of fracture? In short, this highly-informed sample could hardly be considered representative of the general patient population. Further, the trial grants GPs a degree of flexibility that would make its outcomes exceedingly difficult to analyse. Concerned less with whether the trial sufficiently resembled the 'real clinic' and more with the legibility of scientific proof, GPs might misdiagnose patients, or worse, recommend a therapeutic regimen, such as Hormone Replacement Therapy (HRT), that was no longer considered front-line treatment for osteoporosis.

While acknowledging the legitimacy of these concerns, the trial's principal investigator (PI) maintained that the value of the evidence generated about the screening program was directly related to the impact of the study's findings on practice. In his response to the funding committee's review, the PI defended the trial's design on two key grounds. First, he argued that if participation in the trial inspired volunteers to seek clinical advice about osteoporosis, this alone would demonstrate the effectiveness of the screening program. Further, a more proactive research sample might be more likely to modify poor health habits, comply with

---

12   They will receive what is described by the protocol as 'usual care', which, in essence, denotes no proactive involvement whatsoever. Because a control patient's self-reported risk assessments will not be read, GPs will probably only see a patient when she fractures a bone (Lee Shepstone, interview, 21st May 2005).

the GP's treatment advice, and thus, generate more conclusive evidence about the value of a policy of treatment that combines clinical examination with screening. Rather than an obstacle to experimental rigour, the PI argued that the volunteer bias introduced by the self-assessment forms and information packet would reinforce the evidentiary context of the trial by narrowing the distance between trial and practice. Thus, the trial participants would demonstrate the beneficial effects of the program by acting as functional elements of the program itself. Their relationship to patient population would not be merely epidemiological; the pragmatic clinical trial would secure the representative nature of the research sample by coordinating the DEXA scan with patients' health-seeking behaviours.

Second, the PI stressed that the 'sample' included both patients and GPs. The GPs are integrated within the trial's design, not as gatekeepers of a patient population or as executers of a research project, but as part of the intervention and its potential beneficiaries. The team framed variations in GP clinical practice as a problem of information, rather than one of clinical uncertainty. In the same way that pamphlets would educate patients about the management of their disease, a sufficiently detailed protocol would inform GPs about current standards of care, changing their behaviour to improve their clinical practice. The changes initiated by the experimental context to GPs' practices and patient behaviours render moot the accuracy of its depiction of the clinic. What makes the pragmatic trial convincing as a demonstration of effectiveness, is its potential to animate clinical relations, and thereby generate better performance.

The Demo and Participant Publics

In her analysis of trials conducted in the field of cardiovascular disease, Catherine Will describes how researchers incorporate elements of the clinic into their experimental designs in order to enhance the applicability of the results (Will, 2007). Here too, the representative work of the SCOOP trial is not simply mimetic: clinical complexity is resembled so that it may be effectively managed (Armstrong, 2002; Berg, 1997). The funding committee's criticisms of the trial focused on whether or not it could *demonstrate* the effectiveness of its intervention. That the screening program would work was never questioned; its benefits to practice inhered in the diagnostic consistency it promised to generate. It was the steps taken by the design to standardise and order the clinical context that convinced the committee to fund the trial. Thus, the social value of pragmatic fact is keyed to the ordering of clinical practice *in the future*. The practical and prospective endpoint marshals together local domains – the home, the GP's office, the PCT – in the interests of producing quality science. In this sense, the SCOOP trial is not only model of practice – in the sense of a *demo* proving the possibilities of a reality, yet to be actualised (Barry, 2001: 178) – by extending the experiment across clinical and domestic domains, it also creates the conditions for its actualisations.

The public dimensions of experimentation have been a focal topic in the sociology of science and technology (Barry, 2001; Collins, 1988; Latour, 1988; Marres, 2009). For instance work of actor network theorists like Michel Callon, Bruno Latour and John Law have approached experiments as events, whose occasion serves to mobilise resources, interests and support gathering of resources and actors to support claims of truth of effectiveness (e.g. Callon, 1986; Latour, 1988; Law, 1987). What is critical to that understanding is that a public demonstration involves much more than the introduction of scientific facts and technological artifacts into society, but rather a reformatting of society to accommodate and validate new objects. In the cases these authors describe, demonstrations of technologies in public places – on TV and in museums – bring the public in as both audience and participants. Because they involve human participation, clinical experiments add a socio-material dimension to this publicity. The demonstration becomes an occasion for the public to become a user – to involve themselves in the technology through personal and embodied interaction (Marres, 2009).

In the case of the SCOOP trial, that process of integration is particularly intimate, in that it extends diagnostic practice from the clinic to the home. The domestication of technoscientific entities is not a straightforward process of securing public involvement; it requires, to borrow a phrase from Moreira, 'complex forms of articulation work in establishing and maintaining connections between the new technology and those already entangled with users' identities and practices' (Moreira, 2008: 109). To some extent then, the effectiveness of the program to reduce osteoporotic practices depends upon the degree to which patients will be able and willing to entangle diagnostic scales with other daily measures to enhance wellbeing. But as an instrument of publicity, the trial manages that uncertainty by incorporating GPs in the management of diagnosis, who are, much more so than the patients, the key actors in ensuring the workability of the scan within a program of treatment. GPs' clinical knowledge about the risks of osteoporosis, thus, mediates the process through which diagnostic techniques find their way into the home.

In the following section, I describe another pragmatic trial that draws across fields of everyday practice to achieve relevant and robust scientific outcomes. However, while the boundary between SCOOP's experimental model and clinical reality was stabilised within an institutional framework, the provision of primary care in the UK's NHS, in this case, the demo is circumscribed to the private house. This domestic limit is somewhat surprising, as the persuasiveness of its demonstration makes assertive claims on global health policy. However, the context of research is fragmented; the international configuration of actors that fund and direct the trial do not cultivate links to those responsible for national health policy or those involved in health care delivery. In this instance, the local relationships generated and managed through the experiment serve only the ends of proof. Because the trial lacked an administrative framework to extend participants' involvement into public good, its strategies of contextualisation became an expression of its ethical commitment to the participant population. In short, this context of research could only yield a temporary contract – and not a deeper commitment to any future interactions between science and society.

STOPMAL (Screening homes TO Prevent MALaria)

In the innovation-centred world of malaria research, STOPMAL ran against the grain. The study investigated the effectiveness of mesh screens to reduce the number of mosquitoes entering the house. Concerned with methods of vector control, STOPMAL's proposal referenced scientific work from the early part of the century, when malaria interventions formed part of integrated environmental management and social engineering. Like the DEXA scan, in some settings the effectiveness of mosquito-proofing as a preventative measure is uncontested; improvements in low-income housing are commonly thought of as the deciding factor in the elimination of malaria in North America and Europe (Fullerton and Bishop, 1912; Lindsay, 2002; Orenstein, 1912; Schoenfeld and White, 1984; WHO, 1942). But though the use of screens in domestic houses speaks to conventional wisdom, in today's evidence-based climate, these reports are regarded as merely anecdotal.[13] STOMPAL was intended to address those contemporary demands for rigorous assessment, by trailing the effectiveness of screens using a large sample population and a double-blinded, controlled, randomised design. 'If we pull this off,' the principal investigator (PI) explained, 'we should be able to demonstrate, beyond a shadow of a doubt, that good quality housing can dramatically decrease disease burden.'[14] That success had political implications: demonstrating the screen's incontrovertible protective-power could refocus policy attention on simple – rather than sexy – public health strategies.

STOPMAL's sample population included the residents of 500 houses in Farafenni town and the neighbouring peri-urban villages, in upcountry Gambia. The protocol stipulated a three-arm intervention, involving 200 houses with screens hung across their ceilings; another 200 fitted with screens on their windows, eaves, and doors; and 100 left as a control. Compared to the rest of the country, only a small number of Farafenni families used bednets, despite the fact that during the rainy season, malaria rates were relatively high.[15] The PI believed the combination of low bed

---

13 With the notable exception of Angel Celli who, at the end of the 19th century, recorded the incidence of malaria in workers and their families along the railways near Rome. Though it did not conform to RCT methodology, his study illustrated a dramatic difference between those whose houses were screened from those who were not (Lindsay et al. 2003).

14 Matt Kirby, personal communication, 15th May 2007.

15 In Farafenni and its environing, insecticide treated nets are only used in roughly 30% of the households, while malaria rates are about 0–166 infective bites per person per rainy season. This number presents a dramatic decrease following the introduction of bed nets in the country.

net use and seasonal transmission would facilitate the detection of a statistically significant difference between intervention and control. But further, these contextual features promised high levels of acceptability. Where mosquito-bites present only a mild nuisance, people tend to prefer interventions that are less obtrusive; designed with local architectures in mind, the PI hypothesised screens would present a far more attractive – and ultimately more protective – option than a net. He anticipated great experimental returns: at the end of two years, the PI expected to see an almost 80% reduction in the number of mosquitoes entering houses and a similar drop in the prevalence of anaemia in children, as a proxy for malaria infection.[16]

Needless to say, fitting 400 houses with screens was a time-consuming project, requiring considerable human and material resources. Wood had to be shipped from the coast, concrete bought in Senegal, and fly-screening – shipped from Holland – cut into strips and stitched together by a tailor in Farafenni. In addition to the five fieldworkers employed by the trial, the principal investigator hired two teams of carpenters to build and hang screens. Even after narrowing the selection criteria to include only small mud houses with thatched roofs, household architecture varied widely. When installing screens, the field team had to widen doors with machetes or resise windows on the spot.

Maintaining comparable uniformity between houses enrolled in the trial posed an even greater challenge. The PI and his research team had to run constant checks to ensure the screens had been adequately fitted and that there were no gaps. Ceiling screens, weighed down by thatch and mud falling from the roof, were re-hung and mended. Doors, initially secured with a bungee cord, were refitted with latches after villagers complained that children were getting their fingers caught. Moreover, the houses were hardly made of durable stuff; as STOPMAL progressed the PI had to recruit a number of masons from the village to mend holes as brick walls cracked and crumbled. 'We don't screen houses,' he said. 'We fix walls, cement eaves, sand windows and reframe doorways. You'd think I was in the house-building business.'[17]

In light of the intensive construction and reconstruction activities, it is tempting to emphasise the transformative work required to aggregate these domestic places into a single scientific space. It is important to note, however, that these houses are experimental products. First, their layout was the product of colonial experiments in social and environmental management, their ethnic groupings and numbers reflect European conceptions of rural development (Bonneuil, 2000).[18] But more immediately, these villages were the objects of international

---

16   Children were selected because they are most at risk from anemia in this population, which is deemed a good proxy for malaria because it is the most frequent case of deaths.

17   Matt Kirby, personal communication, 10th June 2007.

18   In his analysis of colonial developmental projects, Bonneuil argues that resettlement schemes organised around the introduction of pump-irrigated rice cultivation not only served the purposes of environmental and population management, but also to produce aggregative data for scientific experimentation and analysis (Bonneuil, 2000). In other

medical expert knowledge. Extending 32 kilometres east and 22 kilometres west of Farafenni town, the Farafenni Demographic Surveillance System (FDSS) was one of the first large scale projects conducted from the UK Medical Research Council's (MRC) upcountry research station. The FDSS continues to collect data on 40 villages, comprised of anywhere from 400 to nearly 2,000 inhabitants. Over the years, the FDSS records have provided the starting point for several research projects, its villages the sites for trials and fieldworkers, who live in the villages and are paid annually by the MRC to facilitate recruitment (Geissler et al. 2007). Before recruitment began, the principal investigator used FDSS data to locate eligible houses and to ensure a representative sample. When a house was entered into STOPMAL, its four-part identification code 4:7:31:01 (Village 4: block 7: compound 31: house 1) not only identified it as part of the trial, but located it within the broader geography of experimental practice. Many houses already had numbers painted on them, black-stencilled reminders of the studies that had come before.[19]

Working with a population familiar with research presents clear advantages. In this case the data and contacts made through previous studies, allowed for some shortcuts in enrolment and sensitisation. However, that experimental intimacy also presents challenges. The MRC has been present in The Gambia since 1947, and is now the UK's major research enterprise in a developing country. In recent years, the MRC has expanded upcountry, building field stations in more remote sites, like Farafenni. As research projects have come and gone, providing little in the way of long-term benefits, many Gambian communities have grown wary of the MRC presence in their villages. This distrust is often articulated by rumours that the MRC steals blood and sells it to rich white patients abroad.[20] In their investigation of mothers' engagement with a Pneumococcal Vaccine Trial in the country, Fairhead, Leach and Small (2006) emphasise the precarious nature of the choice to enrol in research: while 'being with the MRC' entitles participants to free medications it also renders them vulnerable to blood-theft. Rather than evidence of a failure to understand medical practices, or alternatively, an articulation of the occult, rumours of blood-stealing are here understood as reflective of the different economies involved in the production of knowledge. 'Joining involves transactions' (2006: 1117); the giving of blood samples and the receiving of therapeutic care

---

words, homes were intended to improve legibility for governance but also disseminate new forms of labour. The question then becomes not how the private spaces are made public, but the different ways in which these spaces have been produced as a public experiment over time.

19   For instance, the Pneummoccal vaccine trial conducted from 2001–2004 throughout the upper half of Gambia, spray-painted numbers on the sides roughly 25,000 houses.

20   Evidence of resistance to medical research has been gathered across Africa: in recent years, scientists have been accused of Satanism, remote blood sucking, and the theft and subsequent resale of African blood (Geissler and Pool, 2006).

is inextricably embedded in the power imbalances and inequalities attendant to global medical sciences and bioscience industry.

Rumours of blood theft are most frequently associated with for studies that require the taking a significant amount of venous blood (e.g. vaccine trials). However, midway through the first year of the STOPMAL, participants started refusing to allow fieldworkers entry to their houses. According to rumours, the light-traps, hung during the night, were being used to collect blood from mosquitoes, which would then be extracted and pooled at the lab, before ultimately being sold. Members of the field team were quick to dismiss the notion that villagers actually believed this convoluted conspiracy. Instead, they saw the rumours as an articulation of their dissatisfaction with the project and offered several competing theories as to its cause. Some thought that in randomising by house (rather than compound or village), had generated some bad feeling when villagers felt they were being treated unequally. Others suggested that the problem stemmed from the behaviour of a young fieldworker from the coast, whose well-educated demeanour and urban clothes had made him unpopular among some participants. The field supervisor cited animosities between two of the leading women in one of the main villages, one of whom had been instrumental in securing support for an earlier trial in that location. Adequate steps had not been taken to appease the other woman before the latest research went ahead and now she was stirring up trouble with her supporters. Whatever the reason, it was clear that the community was unhappy with the way research was being conducted.

To keep participants from withdrawing, the PI held a series of meetings in participant villages. Meetings were conducted at the gathering place in each village's centre – the *bantaba* – and were extended to the whole community, not just those enrolled in STOPMAL. To the assembled crowd, the PI, would reiterate the purpose of the trial, placing particular emphasis on the connection between mosquitoes and malaria. He would then proceed to hang the light trap from a tree and, after switching it on and off, pass around its battery to make clear how it worked. His offer to answer any questions about the device or the project was generally met with little more than nods. At the conclusion to the meeting, the PI announced his promise to screen the houses of those participants who had been allocated to the control arm with whatever kind of screening they would prefer.

The senior fieldworker, who acted as translator, consistently downplayed the significance of the trap in these presentations. Instead he emphasised the duties of participation and maintaining the long-term relationship between Gambia and the MRC. His translation of Matt's careful description of mosquito feeding behaviours was a call to arms: 'we Gambians must work together to see this project through. The MRC has been helping poor people of the Gambia for a long time, it is now up to us to take charge and see that work like this continues.'[21] Participation was a privilege – staying in the trial and following the demands of the protocol, was something the village owed the MRC. Moreover, proactive involvement would lead to future

---

21   Pate, Bah, community meeting, 27th July 2007.

benefits. The field supervisor stressed that if they performed well – maintaining their screens, presenting their children when they needed to have their fingers pricked – they could expect more projects from the MRC. Though they entailed responsibilities, these projects always came with amenities, such as free health care, jobs and even, as in this very special case, structural improvements on their houses.

These public demonstrations not only served to persuade the participants of the safety of a mosquito trap (which admittedly, might not have ever been in doubt) but more important, they also garnered support for STOPMAL. Across the villages, fieldworkers noticed a greater overall enthusiasm about the screens, which in many cases, had been decorated, repaired and even, improved. One mother ingeniously stitched Velcro along the seams of the ceilings screens so that fallen thatch could easily be removed and swept away. Further – and this for the PI constituted a major gain –the participant's accommodation of the screens was reflected in their domestic habits. In the Gambia, doors are open left open as a gesture of trust – a practice, which poses obvious drawbacks for the effectiveness of screen doors. After the demonstrations, fieldworkers found fewer houses whose screen doors had been propped open by rocks.

So what do we make of these efforts to integrate the context into the processes of assessment? On one hand, it is clear that the transformative potential of the trial was only realised after the long-term commitment of the MRC was reaffirmed to the community. The fieldworkers believed that STOPMAL was a 'good trial' because it had made communities more attentive to their home environments. Indeed, focus group discussions conducted at STOPMAL's conclusion indicated that the intervention ultimately proved quite popular. Participants whose houses had been hung with screen-ceilings claimed that their floors were much cleaner; those whose houses had been fixed with screened windows and doors found that they were much cooler. At the end of discussions participants thanked the PI warmly: STOPMAL had been the best MRC 'project' that they had ever been involved with. They then proceeded to show him where their screens needed fixing, the edges along the wall where the mortar had crumbled and the hinges that had lost their screws. Out of funds and out of time, the PI could only give out the name of the two town carpenters, who, he anticipated, after the conclusion of the trial would need the work.

Social Contracts and Public Costs

The results of the STOPMAL trial were extremely positive; screening houses led to a significant reduction both the number of mosquito and the levels of anaemia, even in instances were screened doors were not kept fully closed, and the results were published in *The Lancet* (Kirby et al. 2009). A comment piece from two parasitologists at the US Centres for Disease control (CDC) introduced the paper. Yet after expressing enthusiasm at the return of vector control policies, 'after many years in the proverbial wilderness', they proceeded to question the contemporary feasibility of the strategy:

> Despite the extremely positive results observed in the study by Kirby et al.,
> there are several barriers to surmount before house screening is given the same
> priority as interventions such as LLINs or IRS for malaria control programs.
> Perhaps the greatest barrier to wide-scale implementation of house screening
> will be the question of who pays for it (Gimming and Slutsker, 2009: 954).

Considering the billions ploughed into malaria research annually, balking at the
10 dollars required for full screening seems rather unfair. But the key question of
course, is *who*. A large scale-screening project would certainly gain little support
from commercial partners. The technocratic focus of malaria research on new
vaccines, pharmaceuticals and insecticides that integrate advances in synthetic
biology, produce opportunities for intellectual property or expanding markets.
While perhaps part of an integrated approach, mosquito-proofing housing does not
secure the prize of eradication, put forward by the Gates foundation. To echo the
PI, once the project began house-screening it looked less like scientific innovation
and more like home-construction.

So it is the public who will pay. The success of screens is not only a question
of acceptability, but also of upkeep – people need not only to accommodate
the technology into their daily lives but also to maintain it. Using the home as
a platform, STOPMAL distributed the work and costs of disease control across
different actors – it rescaled malaria from a global disease to a national health
problem. However, in the absence of a public health infrastructure, the costs of
prevention fell squarely on the private household. As the sole focus of a public
health intervention, the homeowner is a problematic cost-absorber. As the
comment piece suggested 'contentious debate between those advocating free nets
and those advocating market-based approaches is likely to resurface should house
screen be strongly advocated for malaria prevention' (ibid. 996). That debate
would be further complicated by the lack of homogeneity of the houses, as well as
uncertainties about how much screening material would be needed and who could
afford installation.

The PI was not surprised by this muted reception. From rather early on his
research, he became convinced that screening did not make practical sense in The
Gambia. After years of working in and on them, he knew houses were simply not
sturdy enough. How then could they justify the cost of an intervention intended
to last three to five years, when the house walls would crumble after two? The
PI could see that screening houses would be a worthy recommendation for army
barracks or for more developed urban areas, for instance, in Tanzania. But for The
Gambia, screens would have to wait until the buildings were made to last.

Conclusion

In drawing these two trials together, I have outlined how the institutional location
of science shapes its social value. SCOOP and STOPMAL share an investigative

aim: to measure the effectiveness of existing technologies within fields of everyday practice. On one hand, that task involves tactics of integration: doorways are sized to fit mesh screens and patients are educated to enable the efficient use of DEXA scan. On the other, these demonstrations require public accommodation: Gambians agree to close their doors and mend holes in netting and GPs alter their practices to a particular version of osteoporosis. This methodological interaction between research and the context simultaneously strengthens the persuasiveness of its claims and enhances its impact on practice. The question the comparison raises is the scale at which the context of research operates. As public experiments, these trials present examples of how the social is reconfigured to absorb innovations (Marres, 2009); but for how long does the reconfiguration take hold and for whom?

In the context of the UK's National Health Service (NHS), where medical evidence is used as the basis for policy decisions, clinical science and the management of public health are intimately connected. As a vehicle directed towards both assessing therapeutic effectiveness and justifying health expenditure, the clinical trial address economic and practical considerations specific to the UK health environment, situating facts within the structures of government policy. Further, by participating in a trial as a patient-citizen, the public orient and exercise jurisdiction over health care interventions. The value of research can be understood in terms of its epistemological gains: the outcomes produced through clinical research will feed back into society through the development of policy and a contribution to scientific knowledge. The pragmatic clinical trial, by internalising the social effects it wishes to make, speeds that process.

The Gambia, in contrast, lacks an administrative framework to link processes of knowledge production to those of modernisation – what Anthony Giddens calls 'looping effects' (Giddens, 1991). While evidence generated through international research projects may eventually help guide health policy, its immediate epistemological benefits (the publication of papers, the advancement of scientific careers and the enhancement of research programs) ultimately short-circuit the experimental context. The domestic context integrated by STOPMAL does not represent a national public, but rather a sample of a pathological geography circumscribed by the 'tropics'. The persuasiveness of its evidence ends with a high profile publication; mosquito-proofing houses become a theoretical privilege for those might be able to afford it. Like SCOOP, STOPMAL addressed issues of scarcity: using local materials and labour, the PI aimed to demonstrate how malaria can be adequately controlled through limited resources. But whereas SCOOP drew upon the UK's NHS as a distributive mechanism, the costs of disease management in The Gambia were devolved directly to the public.

'Contexts', Nowotny, Gibbons and Scott suggest, 'function as a resource and a support that the environment offers to those who find themselves in it; but in turn, an individual or social group must posses the capabilities to perceive and use it' (Nowotny et al., 2003: 256). In western contexts, strategies of public engagement are built into policy processes, have evolved within particular institutional cultures, and articulate specific political imaginaries (Lezaun and

Soneryd, 2007). In contrast, the primary way in the African research context has been made visible is through ethical dialogue. Beyond new moral vocabularies to encompass the dynamics of 'international relations' and the needs of 'whole populations', expanding the ethical milieu has involved mechanisms to elicit a public voice, and indeed, bring specific public forums into being. But where population health is a matter of international and nongovernmental intervention, rather than national politics, these collaborations lack an institutional location to provide the necessarily links between research, policy and practice (Black, 2001; Cooke and Kothari, 2001, Lariumbi, 2008). The context, in short, is an unstable and temporary product of research.

Coordinating a context-specific research agenda requires a rich conceptualisation of the range of actors involved in health care practice. While stressing the social impact of experimental practice, research ethics have traditionally elaborated that impact with regards to specific participants. Recent efforts to expand that conversation to the social value of research tend to understand value as an aspect of the epidemiological relevance of a research question. The contexts in which these pragmatic trials operate are linked with public health: value is generated through the careful alignment of scientific and civic epistemologies.

Taking inspiration from an empirical pragmatics, one way to increase the traction of trials like STOPMAL would be to fix attention on firming up the institutional landscape within which science is carried out. The MRC has the potential to stabilise that context; a long time presence in the therapeutic landscape it mediates the interaction between science and public. However, because it is orchestrated around the trial, the potential of that social contract is constrained by experimental time-frames. The form of commitment is a promise of upcoming projects for which communities remain perpetually 'prepared' – a future that is becoming increasingly uncertain. Though no one knew it then, STOPMAL was to be the last trial hosted in Farafenni. In the February 2009, the staff of the station was informed that MRC head offices in London had shifted its investments in The Gambia to support regional collaborations across West Africa. In addition to closing Farafenni, over the next five years, the MRC will cut The Gambia's medical research budget in half. The rationale – at least the one articulated publicly – is to create the opportunity to conduct multi-centred studies on a greater number of people and thus, enhance the quality of research and the speed at which it is conducted. As one might expect, this plan has not been well received by Gambians, who feel betrayed by the MRC, from whom they had expected a longer commitment. In this instance, as elsewhere on the continent, widening the context to achieve 'greater' relevance may work in the opposite direction, dematerialising the concrete circumstances for public goods to take hold and loosening the structures of social accountability.

Chapter 8

Trial, Trial, Trial Again: Reconstructing the Gold Standard in the Science of Prostate Cancer Detection

Alex Faulkner

Introduction

The study of the implications of detecting the presence of prostate cancer in the male population has become a worldwide medico-scientific endeavour since the early 1990s. Among cancers, prostate cancer is one of the most prevalent and rates of mortality are exceeded only by lung cancer (Cancer Research UK, 2009). It has a high public profile, thanks to media attention to a succession of celebrity sufferers. The question of whether to introduce mass screening programmes, like those in existence for breast cancer and cervical cancer, has been high on the healthcare policy agendas of most of the advanced industrialised countries for many years. This chapter outlines the main dimensions of the controversy over prostate cancer detection in the UK, focussing on scientific-technological uncertainty around population screening, and the ways in which society has responded to (and constructed) the screening issue through scientific medical research in various forms. Indeed, the social and technical extension of the science developed to investigate the issue is the central theme of the chapter. This includes large scale clinically-based trials, 'health services research' in quality of life, and qualitative medical sociology. The chapter shows how the political and scientific development of the detection issue have been implicated in methodological innovations in the production of scientific healthcare knowledge via clinical trials and associated studies, and discusses how these developments contribute to and refract wider dynamics of civil society's apprehension and management of disease risk and uncertainty.

The question of whether to introduce mass population screening programmes raises difficult ethical concerns for public health policy and thus for national governments, which typically seek the strongest possible scientific arguments for such decisions. In cases of scientific uncertainty, such as that to be discussed here, the ethics of intervening in the subjective experience of asymptomatic citizens are confronted, and states' possible role as custodian in the pastoral care of the population is highlighted. Under these circumstances, the 'normal science' of the randomised controlled trial may not be capable of addressing the scientific questions in socially acceptable or methodologically effective ways. This dilemma can be situated in theoretical discussions about both the changing social bases of scientific knowledge and the salience of pastoral care in government. Firstly, challenges to traditional scientific authority through processes of 'contextualisation' have been theorised for example in the concept of mode-2 knowledge production (Gibbons et al., 1994; Nowotny et al., 2001), and to some extent documented in manifestations of citizen science, for example in 'social movements' in health (Brown and Zavestoski, 2005), in the oft-cited example of HIV/AIDS activists in the US (Epstein, 1996), in 'research in the wild' conducted by disease-focused 'concerned groups' (Callon and Rabeharisoa, 2008), and in the mobilisation of lay expertise in science policy participation techniques such as focus groups and citizens' juries. Such developments testify to an opening out of science in which the scientific space becomes more socially permeable. Secondly, the science and practice of disease detection as part of public health policy can be situated in Foucault's discussions of the relationship between pastoral power and the governmentality of the state. In his long historical view, the Western state is seen to have developed techniques of surveillance and intervention in matters of the health, subjective well-being and behaviours of citizens, which have become incorporated into both organised state government activity and into subjective self-care of citizens (Foucault, 1979; 1980). These twin threads of citizen engagement and pastoral power in science will be seen to run through the account offered in this chapter of the evolving science, trials and knowledge practices of prostate cancer detection.

Historical examples show how cancer clinical trials have become embedded in the innovation processes of medical practice over the last half-century (Keating and Cambrosio, 2007). Particular implementations of healthcare science such as the clinical trial may re-arrange social relations, technologies, biological entities and new sociomedical participants. This chapter draws on the concept of 'configuring the user' to examine how the state has involved itself in shaping the experience of citizens who may or may not be at risk of prostate cancer and its detection. The role of the state in configuring users – here citizens, potential patients – has been said to be neglected in science and technology studies (Rose and Blume, 2003). Scientific experiments built into the world of medical and public health practice can be understood in similar ways to those of conventional physical laboratories. The concept of the laboratory as an 'enhanced environment' (Leigh Star, 1991) is useful in highlighting the ways in which science selects and constructs magnified representations of its objects, and shows that an experiment can exist across a range of people, technologies, measurement methods, resources, time periods and institutional organisations, as clinical trials do. Thus this chapter considers the inner workings of healthcare science including experimental trials, giving an example in which its conventional rules and institutional forms are stretched. The reflexive examination of these inner workings can be seen both to construct and respond to broader sociomedical trends.

The provision and consumption of health services is increasingly subjected to the scientific regimes of the clinical trial, transforming healthcare more and more into something resembling a massive array of distributed experimental laboratories (Faulkner, 1997). Recent policy developments in the UK have been explicitly directed toward enhancing the availability of patients to clinical trials, presented as an opportunity for as many patients as possible to take part, through a 'comprehensive' Clinical Research Network, part of the UK Clinical Research Collaboration (UK CRC, 2010). As this book testifies, however, having reached the pinnacle of clinical knowledge creation, the randomised controlled trial (RCT) has now become the object of attention and criticism from a wide variety of perspectives. Of particular importance to trials in prostate cancer detection, as this chapter illustrates, are issues of patients' 'preferences' and of clinical equipoise, the latter referring to the long-established ethical principle that a trial comparing interventions must not be undertaken unless one intervention appears no better than the other, according to the current state of scientific knowledge. The radical re-engineering of the RCT has become a major project of healthcare science itself, as well as of healthcare policy and the various strands of social analysis represented in this book. In this re-evaluation the RCT is emerging as more fragile than might have been expected. Nevertheless, the picture generally is one of adaptation, development and methodological innovation, rather than of abandonment. The case of prostate cancer detection described here illustrates some of these trends.

The chapter draws on a wide variety of sources, including medical and epidemiological research and commentary; surveys of the use and interpretation of the prostate cancer blood test and treatment options by health professionals; interviews with healthcare scientists; public domain testimonies of patients; healthcare policy documents, and archive materials.[1] The author participated in the UK's national Health Technology Assessment (HTA) research programme both as researcher and scientific administrator during the 1990s. The chapter starts with a discussion of the evolution of UK policy in this field, before going on to describe how the scientific exploration and construction of the detection issue has developed. It then touches on the relationship between information and awareness of prostate cancer detection issues in relation to the scientific study of 'quality of life', before concluding with a theoretical discussion of how the development of RCT science can be understood as configuring users through sociomedical uncertainty and the governmentality of the state.

---

1 The main archive used was the Centre for History of Evaluation in Health Care (CHEHC) at Cardiff University, which holds the papers of Sir Miles Irving, the first Chair of the Standing Group on Health Technology in the UK, the body which launched the UK national Health Technology Assessment programme. It also holds papers of Archie Cochrane.

The Policy Problems of Prostate Cancer Detection

The recent history of the relationship between the science and policy of prostate cancer detection is tortuous. Underlying these variations is an extreme degree of scientific uncertainty, which concerns both the value of the PSA test (prostate-specific antigen, a blood test) as predictor of progression of slight signs of the disease ('localised', i.e. organ-confined disease), and the comparative effectiveness of the three major established approaches to therapy: surgery ('radical prostatectomy'), radiotherapy and a 'wait-and-monitor' approach which goes by a number of different medical names. The crucial policy question of whether to introduce population screening programmes hinges largely on the response to these uncertainties. Much of the apparent increase in the rates of prostate cancer over the last twenty years has been attributed to increasing use of the PSA test. It has been clear that widespread use of it by medical practitioners can lead to over-diagnosis, resulting in further invasive clinical investigations and higher levels of radical treatments than might be warranted; nor does a negative result definitely exclude a cancer diagnosis in all cases (Oliver et al., 2001).

The professional specialty most concerned with the PSA and prostate cancer detection issue is urology. In the late 1990s the British Association of Urological Surgeons (BAUS) had produced recommendations to constrain use of the PSA test. A working group stated that 'the unthinking use of PSA, especially in elderly men where it causes distress and anxiety, must be prevented. The role of urologists must be to cooperate with colleagues in other specialties to prevent totally inappropriate investigation... and to ensure that in other circumstances PSA testing is only carried out after appropriate counselling' (Dearnaley et al., 1999). It was clear that policy makers and professional activists feared uncontrolled diffusion of testing – with some reason. A few years later, the government's own cancer tsar regarded the test as already widely diffused in practice, with disastrous effects: 'use of the PSA test is swamping urology and radiotherapy services' according to the Government's 'cancer tsar' (UK newspaper report, 2006).

In the early 2000s prostate cancer was deemed to be of sufficient importance for the government to set up a national Prostate Cancer Risk Management Programme. This put a premium on issues of information provision, including, for example, issuing guidance to all GPs in the country on how to deal with men seeking a PSA test. This and other NHS policy increasingly suggested that patients should be given more information about the test, the implication being that this would limit its use. In 2002, the National Institute for Health and Clinical Excellence (NICE) guidance on 'Improving Outcomes in Urological Cancers' stated:

> One recent change to policy was the decision that PSA tests should be available to men who request them, but that they should first be provided with clear information about the test and the uncertainty about the balance of benefits and risks of screening for prostate cancer... Patients should be offered material designed to promote informed choice about PSA tests (NICE, 2002).

Criticism has then focused around the problems of offering this information. In June 2004 the Committee of Public Accounts, a 'public spending watchdog', raised questions about support for male sufferers, in a situation where women were said to constitute the majority of those using self-help groups for advice about the disease, and expressed concern about an allegedly poor scale of provision of counselling to men (Public Accounts Committee, 2005).

The British government's position on these issues has been to invoke the need for 'more research,' both into the development of better diagnostic tests and by supporting a mega-trial of alternate treatments (ProtecT), funded by the national Health Technology Assessment programme, whose development and significance is discussed in detail below. Government Ministers have continued to invoke the need for more, rigorous knowledge:

> The Government are committed to introducing a national population screening programme for prostate cancer if and when screening and treatment techniques are sufficiently well developed ... The Department is supporting the development of screening technology for prostate cancer by having a comprehensive research strategy (Winterton, 2006).

Some MPs found this position unacceptably passive, arguing that current knowledge about the test should still be circulated more widely. MP Fraser in particular pressed the government about the application to prostate cancer of a novel pilot scheme of 'information prescriptions' (Fraser, 2006), a scheme presented by the Department of Health as part of the commitment to helping patients to feel empowered and participate in decisions about their own care.

Thus the level of policy concern about the detection of prostate cancer has been high because of the implications for health and anxiety of men and families, because of the level of uncertainty in the field, and because of knock-on resourcing effects in the healthcare system. The time needed for scientific research has been presented as an interim period, a 'wait-and-see' position actively tied to the promotion of a need for improved provision of evidence-based information to clinicians and to men themselves. The chapter now considers the involvement of this scientific research, and the RCT in particular, in the shifting contours of policy for localised prostate cancer testing and treatment.

Healthcare Science and Localised Prostate Cancer

Starting in 1994, the Medical Research Council (MRC) in the UK sponsored a multi-centre randomised controlled trial of the three main treatment modalities for localised prostate cancer. The intention was to recruit 1,800 men but fewer than forty gave consent to take part. There were several possible reasons, but according to the clinician-researchers' own account 'many consultants were not willing to randomise patients because they felt they were not in a position of individual equipoise with regard to these treatments (despite clear equipoise in the clinical community overall)' (MRC PR06 Collaborators, 2004). This account clearly shows some major ambivalence about the state of the evidence and its applicability in a trial setting. Other consultants were said to be enthusiastic, but 'found that fully informed patients usually decided which of these three approaches would be most suited to them and would not consent to randomization' (ibid.). Thus this failed trial raised key questions about the forms of commitment to RCTs and attitudes to the balance of scientific evidence in the field that both clinicians and patients might have.

Fuelled by instances such as MRC's PR06, the 1990s saw healthcare science communities give ever greater reflexive attention to their own methodologies. Motivations and incentives to take part in clinical trials, and patients' understandings of their participation in them, have all been the subject of research. The earliest studies used qualitative methods, and showed that the experience of clinical trials was not straightforward (Featherstone and Donovan, 1998; Featherstone and Donovan, 2002). Most patients involved in randomised trials were found to engage in some sort of 'struggle' to understand trial design principles in terms of their own everyday beliefs and knowledge. The part played by clinicians, especially in recruiting patients into trials, was also opened up for qualitative investigation. Research included a study that showed that clinicians attempting to randomise patients within cancer trials used quite variable individual methods of providing information and obtaining consent (Jenkins et al., 1999), and another providing evidence of the range of difficulties faced in some cancer trials (Langley et al., 2000). A later 'Strategies for Trials Enrolment and Participation Study' that reviewed over 100 trials, inconclusively attempted to identify factors determining successful and unsuccessful recruitment (McDonald et al., 2006).

During the same period, the NHS policy-oriented Health Technology Assessment (HTA) programme had got under way, and prostate cancer *screening* had been identified as one of the highest priorities in its first research agenda. The HTA programme commissioned two quantitative systematic reviews (Chamberlain et al., 1997; Selley et al., 1997). These reviews considered hundreds of studies of the performance of PSA tests and its variants, and on the basis of them the Department of Health concluded that there was inadequate evidence to support the introduction of mass screening. In the UK, the two systematic reviews gained iconic and controversial status because they were used at the public launch of the national Health Technology Assessment programme. Thus the prostate cancer screening issue was central to the state-orchestrated build-up of the evidence-based movement in medicine and healthcare in the UK. The public message about screening was negative and was received with dismay by many cancer charities and some urological specialists. On the strength of the HTA reviews, the newly-founded NHS Centre for Reviews and Dissemination (NHSCRD), another part of the growing evidence-oriented national healthcare policy infrastructure, produced advice about PSA testing and prostate cancer for all GPs in England and Wales, and for men who requested it. It was clear that the uncertainty confirmed by the

HTA science was to be shared with GPs and with men themselves. The primary advice was that health professionals should discuss with patients the evidence of the risks of prostate cancer, its treatment *and of its detection* via the PSA blood test. In other words, there was a move toward an information-dissemination and 'counselling' mode of shared decision-making. In a telling decision, cancer charities, whose typical stance was seen to be to advocate early detection and thus early interventional treatment, had their requests for their contact details to be included in the NHSCRD publications declined, indicating the strength of the evidence-based opposition to potential over-use of the PSA test.

The HTA systematic reviews, the associated policy guidance and the failure of the MRC-sponsored trial, combined to heighten debate about how an appropriate clinical trial could be designed in order to address the issues of population screening and treatment. The national HTA programme invited proposals for a trial and became embroiled in debate between potential researchers, including teams variously combining cancer research specialists, powerful urological surgeons and emerging health services researchers. The issue of recruitment to any trial was crucial and controversial, as was the appropriate research question. A large scale randomised controlled trial of *screening versus control,* the European Randomised Study of Screening for Prostate Cancer (ERSPC), had been set up in the early 1990s in several European countries.[2] The ERSPC study was designed as a 'screening trial', in other words a comparison between men randomised to dedicated population screening programmes for asymptomatic localised prostate cancer, and men identified opportunistically through the conventional practices associated with presentation with urinary symptoms and the like, with mortality rates as the primary outcome. It was thus a 'pragmatic' trial, making no attempt to standardise across national practices with regards, for example, to the cut-off point determining the positive/negative interpretation of the PSA test, and the treatment options preferred and practised by the medical and surgical professions in each country-site.

In seeking to agree on a UK trial, the Standing Group on Health Technology received a range of conflicting proposals, with varying research questions, study designs and proposed population settings. One of the urologists campaigning for a specific UK trial suggested: 'men found to have cancer as a result of screening are then found to be unwilling to be randomised to deferred treatment having had the test recommended for early detection'; and 'urologists in the UK are more concerned to develop their experience with radical prostatectomy and are unwilling to participate in an RCT'.[3] A survey of oncologists had shown that they

---

2   The study eventually included 182,000 men, and was reported in 2009 in the prestigious *New England Journal of Medicine* (Schröder et al., 2009), concluding: 'PSA-based screening reduced the rate of death from prostate cancer by 20% but was associated with a high risk of overdiagnosis'.

3   Letter to Chair of Standing Group on Health Technology, cc Chair national HTA Screening Panel. From CHEHC archive.

would generally treat with radiotherapy rather than surgery, a more conservative approach (Savage et al., 1997), but there were rapid increases in urologists' preferences for the use of radical surgery in England during the 1990s (Donovan et al., 1999), later confirmed by NHS data that showed an upward trend in actual rates (Oliver et al., 2003). The same urologist opined that 'the only way to recruit men for a trial of treatment would be to promote PSA testing specifically for this end (i.e. to find 'cases'), which would be regarded as unethical by many and is certainly contrary to the CMO's (government's Chief Medical Officer) view'. Another proposal was for a study that would link in to the ERSPC programme. By focusing on screening, this arguably could avoid the need to randomise men to treatments that neither they nor clinicians would prefer.

Nevertheless there was a widespread belief that research was needed to tackle the problem of low recruitment itself, as illustrated by the abandoned MRC trial and other important cancer trials at the time. In the case of prostate cancer: 'Everyone agreed that the treatment trial was required but no one believed it was possible' (interview, director of ProtecT trial). This set of debates led to the formulation of alternative research plans, which, rather than take the ethical and randomisation-based objections at face value, instead turned them into the subject of an empirical feasibility study. This study would assess whether case-finding through PSA testing was in fact acceptable or unacceptable and would also test modes of recruitment and information-giving in an attempt to improve recruitment levels.

This feasibility study was the one eventually supported by the UK's HTA programme, after lengthy deliberations. It was thus accepted that the screening policy issue could not be resolved whilst uncertainty about preferred treatment modality remained, while the ethics and practicalities of appropriate clinical trial methodology themselves became the subject of sustained reflection. In the account of the director of the 'feasibility' study: 'New methodological approaches are required urgently to ... bridge the gap between clinical practice and the need to acquire evidence ... Such approaches need to retain the essential principle of randomisation while incorporating more fully patients' perspectives and preferences' (Donovan et al., 1999). The incorporation of 'patient preferences' here is crucial to the development of the clinical trial as a societally acceptable tool, as well as to the way in which men were to be configured as recipients of the PSA test and potential treatments.

The state-endorsed feasibility study focused particularly on the initial offer of the PSA test. It exemplified the bringing-together of methods of medical sociology with clinical Health Services Research/HTA using 'qualitative methods'. The design of the study necessitated offering the PSA test to several thousand men in order to identify a small number with the disease who might consent to be randomised to one or other treatment. It aimed to assess men's reasons for participation or non-participation, and to take account of men's own preference, if any, for one or other treatment. The 'qualitative methods' used included face-to-face interviews with men, and recording of consultations in which they were able to discuss information about the PSA test, its uncertain meaning and its potential consequences. Furthermore, men were asked to advise on their interpretation and understanding of the information offered to them, and the researchers used this feedback to make revisions to it. There was an explicit ethical concern that men offered the PSA detection test should be 'fully informed' about the test and possible treatment side-effects, the favoured approach being that this should be in the context of professional face-to-face consultation. These consultations were termed 'information appointments', and thus were quite different from the conventional information sheet and consent form used in other RCTs. The study thus examined the feasibility and social acceptability of case-finding via PSA testing amongst a population of men otherwise unaffected by urological healthcare, the conduct and performance of PSA testing in a screening context, men's attitudes to screening, preferences for treatment of localised prostate cancer, and men's willingness to accept randomisation to one or other form of treatment. In the meantime, importantly:

> ... until more evidence accumulates, patients and urologists should use the information available from recent systematic reviews to reach shared decisions about treating localised prostate cancer and provide information that highlights uncertainties about the potential effects of such treatments on survival and quality of life (Donovan et al., 1999).

This argument, echoing that summarised in the policy discussion at the end of the previous section, made a link between the policy guidance derived from the systematic reviews discussed above, and the approach to information provision and clinical consultation in the feasibility study and potential clinical trial. Both promoted a pastoral model of counselling and 'shared decisions', in clinical practice and in the context of the science of a clinical trial itself.

Accepting Uncertainty and Prioritising Preferences

The feasibility study itself encountered early problems. But at a crucial meeting between the researchers and the national Board of the HTA programme in the UK, one of the urological surgeons involved in the study produced a personal account that turned out to be persuasive in continuing the study, revealing much about the way in which conventional medical practice was being challenged by evidence-based uncertainty at that time:

> (he said that) he always accepted the evidence and but when faced with patients it all became rather difficult and... he was a surgeon and he liked doing surgery... he realised now that, you know, that actually how you talk to patients has an impact on what happens to them ... he hadn't believed that he could talk to patients about being uncertain... but he actually, he had actually found it very

refreshing to be able to say that he didn't really know what was the best thing (interview, ProtecT trial director, 2006).

This construction of individual equipoise, showing a turn toward an approach that admits the possibility of shared uncertainty is reminiscent of a number of 'road to Damascus' style accounts of individual conversions to the cause of EBM (e.g. Smith, 1991), and marked a crucial shift in the credibility of this controversial, methodologically challenging study.

The feasibility study eventually became regarded as a success and led to UK government/HTA programme support for a very large empirical research project. Starting in 2001, this is an unblinded randomised control trial to compare treatment strategies for localised prostate cancer (radical prostatectomy, radical conformal radiotherapy, and active monitoring). It is known as the ProtecT trial (Prostate Testing for Cancer and Treatment). It is still current at the time of writing, being conducted in nine clinical centres in three socioeconomically diverse parts of the United Kingdom. The trial involves the offer of PSA blood tests to 120,000 asymptomatic men aged 50 to 69, with the expectation that 2,000 will be detected as having signs of localised prostate cancer. Men are invited to a nurse-led clinic in general practice in which they are given detailed information about the implications of testing for prostate cancer, uncertainties about treatment, and the need for a treatment trial. If the men consent after a period of consideration, blood is taken for PSA testing. Those with abnormal results are invited to undergo further diagnostic testing. Those expressing a preference choose the treatment they wish. A key feature, required by the ethics committee assessing the study design, was that the 'information appointment' would be conducted by a health professional independent of the research team and professionally trained in counselling. The surveillance of participating men continues for 10 to 15 years after the start, collecting data on quality of life, prostate cancer development, treatment outcome, length of life, and cost implications.

In terms of the evolving methodology of the healthcare sciences, it is notable that this trial was stated to combine 'the qualitative traditions of sociology and anthropology, epidemiological and statistical disciplines informing randomised trial design, and academic urology and nursing', and that the study 'contravened conventional approaches by being driven not by the randomised trial design but by the qualitative research' (Donovan et al., 2002a). Regardless of the interpretation that one might give to this allusion to possible power-shifts in the inter-disciplinary and inter-methodological relationships of the different practitioners of the healthcare sciences, one outcome of the methodological innovations claimed here has been to increase recruitment rates of the ProtecT mega-trial from an estimated 30–40%, to 70%: the study 'showed that qualitative research can help overcome otherwise prohibitive recruitment problems' (Donovan et al 2002a). Notably, the increased salience of qualitative sociology/anthropology, which required high-level debate with research policymakers before it made headway, emerged from 'technical' problems of data capture and citizen-patient enrolment.

The ProtecT trial has been extended to allow for a number of innovative sub-studies. One small study using qualitative interview methods was designed to address the question of why men agree or decline to take part in the trial, and highlighted issues of preference and equipoise. Ten of the eleven men who refused randomisation did not find equipoise acceptable, whereas five of the six who clearly accepted equipoise consented to randomisation (Mills et al., 2003). Many of the men had strong feelings about the acceptability of randomisation, and many of those consenting to randomisation nevertheless did so with the proviso that they could choose their preferred treatment if it did not fall to them by chance – an approach the researchers interpreted as offering 'comfort' to the men taking this view (Mills et al., *op.cit.*). Other men felt that the clinicians probably really did have an idea that one or other treatment approach was suitable them individually (Mills et al., *op.cit.*). There was also some indication that the difficulty of the decision-making choice itself could for some be *alleviated* through the randomisation procedure. The authors also note problems for statistical design and analysis of trials in which strong personal preferences for one or other arms might exist (not discussed here). The conclusions emphasise the difficulty that clinicians might experience in shared decision-making consultations with patients: 'the ability of clinicians to convince patients of their uncertainty is crucial' (ibid.). It is clear that such a position may conflict with other aspects of clinical relationships with patients and may be especially problematic where the health practitioner responsible is also the trial recruiter.

The incorporation of 'patient preferences' in the trial itself shaped the image of the potential patient, or 'user' of the PSA test. The ProtecT feasibility study and the main trial position men in several choice-situations such as deciding whether to agree to the PSA test, and whether to contribute to re-designing information provision, linked to issues regarding any potential preference for one or other form of treatment. However, as Mills *et al*'s study demonstrates, choice is not a fixed characteristic of individual personalities or life-situations, but is something that might evolve in interaction with medical and nursing professionals, family and mass media, and the healthcare system broadly. Thus in the ProtecT trial some expressed 'preferences' may have been formed as post hoc rationalisations of participation in the randomisation process. The broad implication of the attempts to grapple with problems of preference and equipoise is that more emphasis will be given to communicating to patients the uncertainty about alternative options, which the ethical concept of equipoise necessitates. However, the adherence of clinicians to belief in equipoise in the case of given trial set-ups is by no means straightforward. For example, clinicians may distinguish between different sorts of knowledge in appraising their position regarding the uncertainty of evidence, and may base their position on some clinical categories of patients rather than others (Tomlin et al., 2007).

A further innovation claimed for the ProtecT trial is that the 'users have been involved in the design and conduct of an ongoing trial' (Donovan et al., 2002b), and a case has been made by the scientists, as noted above, for the *primacy* of 'qualitative research' in this knowledge-generating project, informing the design of the trial, recruitment strategy, and information for participants (Donovan et al., 2002a). Thus this represents a significant departure from the normative model of positivist healthcare science represented by health technology assessment (Williams et al., 2003). Indeed, it would be recognised by many as close to an 'action research' model of the knowledge-generation process, though this is a social science research terminology that this research team has not itself espoused.

Informed Citizens, Choice-Making and the Quality of Life

In the case of ProtecT, alongside the primary trial question of the comparative effectiveness of alternative treatments, questions about men's experience of the PSA test and of the research project itself have been shown to have been crucial. In part, this is because understanding of these issues was deemed to be key to enable the primary trial to take place with any chance of recruiting adequate numbers. But this move toward investigating men's experience also clearly reflects a concern that exposure to the PSA test, or even exposure to information about the PSA test, might itself have some health-related consequences for male citizens and their significant others. Thus men's experience has been the subject of investigation emanating directly from the ProtecT trial (Brindle et al., 2006), as well as other research and information sources (Chapple et al., 2002; Evans et al., 2007; DIPEX; Faulkner, 2008).

This pastoral concern is demonstrated in some Health Services Research projects that have attempted to investigate men's experience of PSA testing using conventional quality-of-life measurement tools such as the Hospital Anxiety and Depression Score and the SF-36, probably the most widely used 'activities of daily living' instrument in worldwide healthcare research. One such study directly linked to the ProtecT trial concluded that the standard health status tools did not capture the effects on men of receiving an abnormal PSA result (Brindle et al., 2006). This is surprising when considered in the face of qualitative accounts provided by men in interviews and personal testimonies such as those in the DIPEX online resource, which show that emotional reactions can be extreme.

Another strand of healthcare science has focused on the effects of 'information' on men's attitudes to undergoing the test, and second on the psychosocial impacts of the test. However, a review of information provision (e.g. leaflets, video, counselling) found a lack of firm evidence. Whilst information provision has been deemed generally to reduce the proportions of men interested in undergoing the test, this was markedly less strong when free testing was offered as part of research projects, resulting in the conclusion that 'considerable caution should be exercised when attempting to draw conclusive links between the role of information in improving knowledge in men considering the PSA test and the relationship between information provision and men's intention to have the PSA test' (Hewitson and Austoker, 2005: 25). The quality of evidence also appeared problematic in the case of the psychosocial impacts of testing. Therefore, conclusions such as 'Prostate cancer screening may be viewed by men as a routine examination, and therefore does not cause significantly large increases in HRQoL (Health-Related Quality of Life) or anxiety levels' (Essink Bot et al., 1998), may not be reliable. Hewitson and Austoker's review is useful in further illustrating the close discursive linkage that was emerging between scientific uncertainty on the one hand and the counselling model of pastoral practice on the other:

> Given that the most uncertainty and lack of conclusive scientific evidence is related to the consequences of having the PSA test (e.g. the benefits of early detection, the effectiveness of prostate biopsy, doubt surrounding the impact that treatment may have on a man's quality of life, etc.) it is vital that men are fully informed of the possible ramifications that having a PSA test may hold (Hewitson and Austoker, 2005).

Supporting this linkage further, amongst the guidance produced by the expert group of the Prostate Cancer Risk Management programme, mentioned in the section on policy above, has been the issue of how to deal with men suffering from LUTS (lower urinary tract symptoms). The following are amongst the conclusions: 'Experts disagree as to whether men with LUTS should "opt-in" or "opt-out" of the PSA test, but all agree about the importance of fully counselling these men about the test implications'; '… until more evidence is available about screening for prostate cancer, active case finding of men with risk factors is not recommended' (Watson et al., 2002). In the absence of clear evidence about men's experience and about comparative treatment effectiveness, therefore, both government policy and scientific commentary have emphasised the model of the informed and counselled citizen and patient.

Conclusion: Reconfiguring and Re-legitimating the Gold Standard

The healthcare science of prostate cancer detection has been conducted at a symbolically important level in the UK, as elsewhere. The primary national UK study, ProtecT, has constructed a novel, worrying, risky, laboratorised evidence-rich sociomedical space. This represents in part a response to the growing concern about the workings of informed consent procedures and healthcare user understandings of clinical trial principles. But it was also deemed necessary to engage in a reflexive investigation of the methodology of the trial itself – turning the spotlight onto the practices underlying the entire knowledge project. Insights developed from men's reactions and understandings of trial principles and information presentation were used to re-design the recruitment process. The enrolment of asymptomatic citizens into long-term healthcare laboratories was accomplished through methodologies which attended to the specific experiences, anxiety, linguistic interpretations, and choice-making practices – preferences – of men. Thus the scientific work of the eventual trial has been informed not only by qualitative methods but has also been framed as a participative methodology, in which 'users' may be seen as beneficiaries of the research process to which they themselves are contributing. Citizens have thus been configured as both subjectivities in, and objects of, the scientific research process, reflecting the twin threads of citizen engagement and pastoral power introduced in the introduction to this chapter.

The move toward a counselling and shared-decision-making model of interaction between men and healthcare systems, and between men and scientific research is evident. Healthcare and science have become engaged and entangled with men's subjective experience outside as well as inside conventionally-bounded medical frameworks. Returning to the notion of 'configuring the user', and the state's participation in this, it can be seen that the science of prostate cancer detection, including large-scale trials and quality of life assessment, mandated by centralised symbolically important state funding, has contributed to constructing citizens as legitimately to be invited to and exposed to asymptomatic testing and to extreme evidential uncertainty. This has been accomplished through a pastoral process of information-sharing and counselling built into scientific investigation, and through participative science drawing on the technical resources of qualitative research methodology. A re-negotiated, attenuated form of societal control persists in these reconfigurations. The information-sharing, preference-accommodating, counselling model has strong echoes with Foucault's analysis of biopower, where self-knowledge and care for oneself are seen as part of the individualising force of governmentality in what he termed 'pastorship' – the 'pastoral modality of power' (Foucault, 1979). The methodological extension of clinical trial methodology has thus produced sociomedical sites in which major societal and power dynamics are inscribed – the urge to citizen involvement; the mediation of the state into custodianship and pastoral care; and diffusion of uncertainty and risk into individual subjectivities. The construction of healthcare laboratories here escapes the confines of the healthcare system itself. Such laboratories create enhanced environments not only for the production of knowledge and containment of uncertainty, but also for the provision of care in society: ultra-informed consent and ultra-counselled deliberation.

Thus we see some signs here of a re-socialisation of modernist science, in which the modes of trial practice – the social worlds of the trial – are being extended and adapted in various dimensions. The developments chronicled in this chapter are in line with the well-known theory of a movement toward 'mode-2' production of knowledge (Gibbons et al. 1994). The mega-trial of prostate cancer detection can be regarded as at the same time a socially and a methodologically 'extended RCT', moving toward more 'socially robust' forms of scientific endeavour (Nowotny et al., 2001). The greater permeability of the scientific space does not mean that knowledge produced there is more certain but that it is more procedurally legitimated. Having seen in the later 20th century a phase in which medical practice was being 'turned into a science' (Berg, 1995), we are witnessing now perhaps a second wave of the progression of scientific medicine in which science in the form of the gold standard clinical trial is being turned into, or at least out toward, a more socially sensitive practice. Through incorporation of techniques of information-giving, counselling and engagement of men in the scientific project, the ethical and pastoral concerns of the state have been brought into closer alignment.

An important question is to identify the conditions which predispose some trials, or sequences of scientific study, more than others, toward these sorts of development. In prostate cancer detection it can be suggested that the extreme level of uncertainty regarding both the performance of the detection test and the relative merits of possible therapies have been key factors, along with the high stakes involved in cancer. High uncertainty and high stakes might be conducive to innovation in knowledge methods and the principles of knowledge production – this might be applicable also, for example, in the well-known case of HIV/AIDS activism in the US (Epstein, 1996). However, an interesting and obvious contrast here is that in the case of prostate cancer detection in the UK there has been no citizen or patient-based activist movement targeting the science, the concerted impetus instead originating more from health policy-makers, clinicians and healthcare scientists.

Whilst the practice of medical population screening is perhaps a quite obvious technique of governmental power (cf. Vailly, 2006), this chapter shows how the scientific study of screening-related practices through clinical trial techniques can be understood in the same way. In this instance, the state advances in order to retreat. In so doing it constructs citizens (configures users) as reflexive self-regulators presented with information that is difficult to resist and which is tied to peculiar forms of advisory care (counselling) in order to be incorporated and coped with in people's daily lives. If the move documented here offers any form of 'salvation' (cf. Coveney, 1998), it is knowledge itself – 'self-knowledge' here being the knowledge of one's position in terms of a medico-governmental risk profile. Knowledge of personal, subjective uncertainty is construed, through the state's collective pastoral custodianship, as a virtue. In this move of directive non-direction, a pastoral science proceeds ambivalently as both medicalising and de-medicalising. In more social philosophical and humanist terms (Deleuze, 2007), the science of prostate cancer detection might be regarded as a site at which liberation and enslavement meet.

Acknowledgments

I thank Jenny Donovan, director of ProtecT, for discussions and information about the ProtecT trial and its associated studies.

Conclusion:
So What?

Tiago Moreira and Catherine Will

In the introduction we framed this book as a series of empirical studies of the contemporary incarnations of the clinical trial. We suggested that this particular form of experiment was facing new methodological, regulatory, and sociological challenges, which are being met with methodological innovation *and* developments in the institutional arrangements for the use of trial data. From this perspective, the chapters of this book provide evidence of the ways in which trials are interacting with shifting political, regulatory and clinical contexts. In the conclusion, we draw on this evidence to ask: so what? What are the implications of this research for clinicians and patients? What are the consequences for a critical understanding of the links between evidence and policy? What, if any, are the lessons learned for health research itself? First however we start with a more basic question about the contribution that ethnography in particular might make to this field.

Why Ethnography?

When organising this volume, we were often drawn to consider the contrast between the research practices described in the chapters and the methodological procedures used by the authors of the chapters themselves. On the one hand, the chapters reported on highly organised, standardised and regulated forms of knowledge production, while on the other, those reports were themselves reliant on inductive, adaptive and often informal methods of data collection and analysis. While this divergence between the methods of science and the methodologies of academic observers of scientific practice has sometimes become the focus of disputes about the authority of science in public life, our attraction to this tension was motivated by our belief that qualitative studies of clinical trials can provide important evidence for the continuing transformation of the RCT that this book aimed to explore.

This interactive relationship between RCTs and qualitative studies has been increasingly recognised. It is now accepted by institutions such as the UK's Medical Research Council that qualitative methods like semi-structured or open interviews or ethnography have an auxiliary function to clinical trial methodology. Indeed, Faulkner (this volume) reports on a trial where qualitative interviews were embraced by researchers to inform trial design by elaborating on patient experiences and perceptions, though this interest was conspicuous by its absence in Dehue's example. Yet such methods are less often seen as valuable in addressing professional practice or beliefs. Our suggestion is that qualitative research can contribute also to understanding the connections, networks, organisations and institutions that are deployed in the production and evaluation of trial evidence.

Here ethnography has something particular to offer. As we suggested in the introduction, the chapters in this book all approach the clinical trial through detailed case-studies, resulting from sustained involvement with the events and interpretations of the case, through direct immersion and/or extensive documentary analysis. As a result, the chapters are rich in empirical detail and conceptual validity, derived from what Jack Katz has labelled analytical induction, where researchers 'simultaneously [look] for an explanation that will fit all the evidence and for a definition of the problem that, without "cooking" or hiding data, makes relevant only the evidence that fits the explanation,' (Katz, 2002: 485). Ethnography is intrinsically exploratory, making a virtue of its flexibility. Analysis, hypothesising and data collection are often intertwined. In accepting this approach to research, the question or questions asked of the data keep changing, and 'at each juncture something more is generated than the answer requires' (Strathern, 2004: xxii). In the RCT, the use of randomisation, blinding and uniform reporting standards seek to reduce the 'bias' that may accompany discretion on the part of researchers or clinicians. In ethnography, the researcher (and it often is an individual working alone) must use their involvement as the means of producing rich and subtle understandings of a local situation. What then could ethnographers possibly have to say to researchers who work through and with the more formal methodology of the trial? We offer three tentative suggestions, which relate to issues flagged in the introduction: the challenges of making RCT data 'relevant' to practitioners or policy makers; potential 'logics of involvement' to draw patients and health care providers into the production and interpretation of evidence; and questions about the public life of trials, particularly their importance for public policy.

Relevance and the Limits of Standardisation

Clinical researchers themselves have a number of strategies for accommodating the unpredictability that is part of clinical practice, so that trial results may be understood as having general applicability. Key among these is the concept of 'effectiveness' as a broader concept than 'efficacy', a move also formalised in the typology of Phase I to Phase IV studies, as well as Intention To Treat analyses. These work powerfully by acknowledging local, individual diversity, but agreeing to 'bracket' it for the sake of interpretation (Will, 2007) rather than trying to account for its features in evaluating the results of any single trial. The authors in this book suggest a different conceptualisation of the relationship between local and universal. Through engagement with places where trial results are produced and interpreted, again and again they reveal the crucial role of local knowledge and work in these processes. Ad-hoc adaptations of method, shifts in the formulation of questions, readiness to alter routine ways of reasoning, all contributed to the processes of 'discovery' in trials as well as in ethnography. In this sense, local everyday practice is not something that can be acknowledged in experimental design only to be set aside in analysis. Rather, as our contributors repeatedly point out, improvisation is also required to help the experiment take place, and has implications for the meanings of its results.

Thus making a trial work scientifically entails attending to a variety of concerns and demands that are normally considered to be extraneous or damaging to research. For Heaven, for example, the problems encountered in enrolling nurses in trial data collection should not be understood as evidence of the recalcitrance of health care professionals, but rather of the difficulties of engaging nurses with standardised educational strategies while attending to the challenges that they face in daily practice. In this case, one might argue that what Heaven sees as an ontological divide between scientists and practitioners is also an epistemological problem where no one could find appropriate formal ways to acknowledge and crucially to share information about the real difficulties of changing clinical practice. Yet in Helgesson's case study a good deal of rather messy work was required to tidy up inconsistencies or gaps in trial data, and in this process the distance between local practices and 'centralised' data management was crucial. Knowledge production relied on an apparent lack of communication. A similar internal mismatch within the trial is also revealed in Timmermans' work where, while the pharmacological comparison in the formal design of the study pointed to a lack of efficacy, the trial can be seen as providing additional *useful knowledge* about the needs and preferences of users of methamphetamine, as well as data on the gaps and insufficiencies of existing services.

A possible response to such findings would be to take them as evidence of flaws in the production of evidence: protocols were not followed strictly, standards were adapted, etc. Method was not respected. We, however, would like to argue that ethnographic evidence of the kind offered here, helps us understand what it takes for clinical trials to produce meaningful data *through* such conditions, and acknowledge the work done to make them happen. Thus the epistemic tensions and conflicts that Heaven, Timmermans and Helgesson identify are integral to knowledge making in clinical trials. To an extent, this is not surprising. Studies of scientific practice in other domains have documented that pragmatic tensions and local constraints experienced and resolved by researchers in their day-to-day working lives become embodied in the production of innovative models, ideals or products (Knorr-Cetina, 1999). Yet, these are rarely recognised as part of scientific practice. The work of coordinating and balancing tensions between professional groups involved in the trial, or research and care, and of making such balances work in local contexts likewise has consequences for the success or otherwise of the clinical trial. Successful trials – those that are actually able to recruit and gather outcome data – are able to adapt methodological standards to local contexts and demands.

What are the consequences of this for the interpretation of trials, for claims about their relevance and importance in the world? Clinicians and policy makers already try to piece together information about the context in which trials were carried out in order to answer these questions. Thus Kelly (this volume) work reveals how the differential reception for two trials was underpinned by the interpretative resources deployed by readers, such that the results of trials conducted in the Gambia were read by other researchers as irredeemably situated, even if they were published in international journals. Will (this volume) documents another 'localisation' strategy used by interpreters of clinical trials linking their results to their commercial context, though it was suggested that the increasing standardisation of trial appraisal might exist in some tension with such collective critique. Could such accounts of the local conditions of knowledge production be complemented by a more positive view of local work such as the one we suggest?

One site where one might draw on such critical, contextualised readings of trials might be in the ethical review and regulation of research. Here ethics committees may do well to acknowledge the ways in which participating in trials may provide forms of care that are valued by patients, rather than seeking to maintain a rigid distinction between relationships for the purposes of research and those inherent in clinical practice (Timmermans, this volume). Furthermore, difficulties of recruitment and retention such as those described by Heaven and Faulkner (this volume) could perhaps be investigated as 'flags' for epistemic weakness, rather than organisational difficulty. While ethical review is currently concentrated on the time before trials begin, reluctance to get involved once the trial is underway should perhaps be taken seriously as a sign of a problem with the trial question or design, as briefly noted in Faulkner's chapter, but only if researchers are then enabled to respond flexibly to the difficulties, rather than given a choice between working to a pre-defined protocol or abandoning the study.

Another site when we might want to account for the 'local' work required to produce evidence comes in the translation between trial data and clinical guidelines or recommendations. In previous work Moreira (2005) has argued that unlike systematic reviewers, guideline-writing groups endeavour to include assessments of the 'acceptability' and 'useability' of recommendations, as well as the robustness of the evidence on which they may be based. Social scientists have proposed that such efforts might form part a 'reflexive health technology assessment' (Webster, 2007). Here both Faulkner and Moreira (this volume) suggest that the production of evidence is increasingly structured by reflexivity and interactions between practitioners and policy makers in order to collectively explore the links between local constructs and standards. Yet much more information on both the acceptability and useability of interventions is generated in the process of carrying out and evaluating trials, but still only briefly, locally, and informally acknowledged (i.e. one could say this information never becomes data). There is more to be done to ground claims to relevance in the experience of research, and acknowledge these issues even in fields that do not spark immediate controversy.

Logics of Involvement

We noted in the introduction the rise of a language of 'involvement' that calls for researchers to find ways to include patients and public in decisions about the design of clinical trials and research questions. Again, methodologists themselves offer some ways forward, including discussions of 'outcomes that matter to patients,' 'research for patient benefit' and patient priorities. We are also increasingly seeing calls for patient-friendly information about trials: for example the UK's Clinical Research Collaborative appears to pay great attention to education about the workings of randomised controlled trials, offering diverse resources to school teachers on their website, and several prominent science journalists also work as advocates for this methodology to the reading public. Efforts such as those charted by Faulkner (this volume) to draw on patient experiences and beliefs in defining appropriate interventions are becoming increasingly common. Yet our contributors map a very diverse set of 'involvements' that accompany clinical research, and point to some of the limits of current models of participation.

Thus Timmermans (this volume) offers data showing that many patients are simply uninterested in the facts of the trial, seeking treatment and/or sympathy but refusing to engage in discussions of research design or results. In some sense, Heavens' (this volume) discussion of professional responses has some similarities with this account: nurses are too busy with managing everyday patients to allocate energy to research on a single intervention for one condition. In contrast Kelly (this volume) describes a situation of 'experimental intimacy' between particular villages in Africa and researchers funded by the UK's Medical Research Council, where research and care is closely and explicitly linked, and participants are actively concerned with the organisation of trials. However such intimacy does not prevent frequent misunderstandings or tensions between researchers, whose involvement is contingent on decisions about funding made far away, and participants, who are much more involved with immediate economic and social problems facing their communities than the knowledge generated through trials. These accounts suggest that there are likely to be considerable difficulties with models of research that demand patient involvement, if particular populations have good reasons not to engage. Non-engagement should be taken seriously, as it denotes dis-articulations between research agendas and patients' needs and ways of life (Moreira, 2006). The most effective involvement will go beyond discussions about the nature of interventions or outcomes, to discuss bigger issues relating to the choice of research question and distribution of care at the end of the trial.

Advocacy by both patient and professional groups appears one way to amplify the patient voice (Callon and Rabeharisoa, 2008), and their increased importance forms a backdrop to both Dehue's account of national depression guidelines in the Netherlands and Moreira's discussion of the alliances emerging in controversy about expensive drugs for slowing the effects of Alzheimer's in the UK. But both also suggest that these patient groups have difficulty being recognised as distinctive and credible voices in a public debate about therapeutic approaches and health priorities. In Moreira's case, this might be linked to the fact that their involvement was limited to the discussion of evidence that already had been produced and standardised, excluding meaningful input about the types of outcomes patients want from health interventions (Chalmers, 1995). As Will and Dehue's chapters make clear there are important gaps between the types of reasoning used to justify therapeutic development and the requirements of clinical practice.

This means that involvement cannot be thought of as 'step' in developing and assessing research with the help of institutional outsiders (usually patients). It requires strong institutional support for communication between clinicians, manufacturers, researchers, patients and policy makers. Rather than seeking to systematically monitor research against standards for public involvement and consultation, these processes might entail shifts in the roles that these groups play in the governance of knowledge and in standard setting (Moreira, 2007). The chapters from both Will and Moreira are illustrative of some of the uncertainties that surround such shifts. In the case of the dementia drugs controversy, professionals emerged as successful advocates, but only to re-affirm clinical autonomy and lines of accountability that exclude non-expert groups. In Will's study, on the other hand, clinicians and researchers were able to join in elaborating zones of uncertainty in an attempt to reduce the ability of pharmaceutical companies to harness research to marketing agendas. However their effectiveness was ultimately in doubt. It was more possible to chart an effect in Faulkner's case, where sharing such uncertainty between doctors and patients helped bring about new research designs *and* clinical practice (indeed, as Faulkner points out, the emphasis on sharing uncertainty in a clinical encounter framed as 'counselling' is a striking contemporary theme, also apparent here in the trials described by Timmermans and Heaven). Social scientists may be able to help map the ways in which such processes could and should contribute to involvement in its widest sense. The chapters in this book identify some of the institutional processes through which involvement is deployed, from the designing of research questions to the evaluation of data. More work is needed to recognise and formally integrate those processes and identify the groups that should be invited into such platforms.

Evidence and Policy

Campaigners for Evidence-Based Medicine (EBM) have on the face of it had startling success in the last two decades, shaping new political debates about 'evidence-based policy making' and setting the RCT at the top of a hierarchy of evidence in increasing numbers of policy areas. Yet they can also seem dissatisfied not only with the failure to implement evidence consistently, but also with the vagaries of public funding for research and the reluctance of governments to take on commercial sponsors in the name of rational policy-making. Many of our chapters focus on questions about the interaction between the governance of knowledge and health care in contemporary societies. Through their detailed accounts of the processes that surround the imputation of authority to data and its transformation into evidence, they provide a rich understanding of the ways in which scientific work is shaped by regulatory and policy frameworks. Again, this was not done to 'denounce' the political character of trials, or undermine the value of evidence in political life. As other researchers have demonstrated, scientific evidence is always produced in the context of diverse political and economic agendas and priorities (e.g. Jasanoff, 2005). Yet our contributors, especially Faulkner, Moreira and Dehue, reveal how policy emphasis on particular types of evidence is still linked to specific forms of health care organisation and delivery.

In Faulkner's chapter, the search for evidence accompanies the elaboration of government interest in health promotion, raising questions about the involvement of the state in such preventive action, even if it can be justified as cost effective. For Moreira, efforts to 'model' responses to particular drugs in order to prioritise resources in a national health service produce new categories of patient, whose relevance is hotly contested by clinicians and patients' families living with the daily challenges of Alzheimer's. And in Dehue's chapter, the focus on pharmaceutical treatments for depression reduces the space to talk about social and familial causes of mental ill health, and the importance of social support for sufferers. In this context, the emphasis by some social scientists on 'public' funding for clinical research (see e.g. Sismondo, 2008; Petryna, 2009) requires more attention. Such statements may lead to confusions between political representation and inclusion in experiments (Epstein, 2007), or fail to assess the ways in which state agendas will have their own effects on the research that may be done.

The drive to cut healthcare costs may prove a powerful counter to commercial efforts to expand pharmaceutical markets, but as is apparent in the UK, interest in preserving industrial activity may appear to limit such effects, while powerful commercial interests are also involved in healthcare provision, especially in the US. Increasing attention is being paid to the problems that result when trial data is not made publicly accessible, but retained as the property of pharmaceutical companies. But we should also draw attention to the trials that are not and will not be done (Will, this volume) and the limitations of the evidence base described above. The reliance on trial evidence in practice and policy risks reinforcing forms of social and economic exclusion with what might be terms an *epistemic exclusion*, as problems and populations that do not come to the attention of academic researchers become locked out of forms of health care that are supported by such research and innovation. Epistemic exclusion is characteristic of societies that are heavily reliant on research and technology. However, while social and economic exclusion have been the concern of public health for many years and are increasingly recognised as an important area of policy, the same cannot be said about the current detachment of certain groups from the collective production of knowledge. Such processes of exclusion are linked to a complex network of factors: the reliance on competiveness in national and international R&D policies (Felt et al., 2007); manufacturers' preference for widely defined product labels; and interactions with other forms of social inequality.

We hope to have shown in this book that the trial works best in collaboration with other knowledge making approaches. This goes beyond a call for interdisciplinarity. Understanding the political and economic contexts in which clinical trials are conducted and reported should help identify creative approaches to knowledge governance. To address the forms of exclusion that the emphasis on the clinical trial appears to have produced, policy makers and researchers should explore what other knowledge forms are appropriate to such unique conditions. Qualitative studies of groups, or case studies of individuals should be considered valuable sources of information in understanding and addressing new forms of exclusion in the evidence-based state.

Conclusions

Three 'mindlines' can therefore be usefully extracted from our book:

1. Information about how clinical trials are organised and carried out goes beyond reporting of methods and is crucial for critical interpretation of evidence.
2. Involvement should not be seen as auxiliary to knowledge production within clinical trials, but embedded in different stages of their design and interpretation.
3. Absence of evidence might be a good indicator of forms of exclusion for which methodologies such as the case study can be more appropriate.

Bibliography

Abraham, J. (1995). *Science, Politics and the Pharmaceutical Industry: Controversy and Bias in Drug Development.* London and New York: Routledge.

Abraham, J. (2007). Drug trials and evidence bases in international regulatory context. *BioSocieties*, 2(1): 41–56.

Abraham, J. and Lewis, G. (2000). *Regulating Medicines in Europe: Competition, Expertise & Public Health.* London: Routledge.

Abramson, J. (2004). *Overdo$ed America: The Broken Promise of American Medicine.* New York: HarperCollins.

Angell, M. (1988). Ethical Imperialism? Ethics in international collaborative clinical research. *New England Journal of Medicine*, 319: 1081–83.

Angell, M. (2004). *The Truth About the Drug Companies: How they Deceive Us and What To Do About It.* New York: Random House.

Armstrong, D. (2002). Clinical autonomy, individual and collective: The problem of changing doctors' behaviour. *Social Science & Medicine*, 55(10): 1771–7.

Armstrong, D. and Ogden, J. (2006). The role of etiquette and experimentation in explaining how doctors change behavior: a qualitative study, *Sociology of Health and Illness*, 28(7): 951–68.

Armstrong, D., Lilford, R., Ogden, J. and Wessely, S. (2007). Health-related quality of life and the transformation of symptoms. *Sociology of Health and Illness*, 29(4): 570–83.

Ashcroft, R. and ter Meulen, R. (2004). Ethics, philosophy and evidence based medicine. *Journal of Medical Ethics*, 30: 119.

Ashmore, M., Mulkay, M. and Pinch, T. (1989). *Health and Efficiency: A Sociology of Health Economics.* Milton Keynes: Open University Press.

Ballard, C.G. (2006). *Presentation on Alzheimers Drugs.* House of Commons, 16 January 2006.

Barry, A. (2001). *Political Machines.* London and New York: Athlone Press.

Baruch, G. (1981). Moral tales: parents' stories of encounters with the health professions. *Sociology of Health & Illness*, 3(3): 275–95.

Bauman, Z. (2007). *Liquid Times. Living in an Age of Uncertainty.* Cambridge: Polity Press.

Begg, C., Cho, M., Eastwood, S. et al. (1996). Improving the quality of reporting of randomized controlled trials: the CONSORT statement. *JAMA*, 276: 637–9.

Benatar, S.R. (2004). Towards progress in resolving dilemmas in international research ethics. *Journal of Law, Medicine & Ethics*, 32: 574–82.

Benatar, S.R., Singer, P.A., and Daar, A.S. (2005). Global challenges: the need for an expanded discourse on bioethics. *PLoS Medicine*, 2(7): e143. doi:10.1371/journal.pmed.0020143

Benatar, S.R., and Fleisher, T.E. (2007). Ethical issues in research in low-income countries. *International Journal of Tuberculosis & Lung Disease*, 11(6): 617–23.

Berg, M. (1997). *Rationalizing Medical Work: Decision Support Techniques and Medical Practices*. Cambridge, MA: MIT Press.

Berg, M. (1995). Turning a practice into a science: reconceptualising postwar medical practice. *Social Studies of Science*, 25(3): 437–76.

Bernard, C. (1865). *Introduction à L'étude de la médecine expérimentale*. Paris: Ballière.

Bero, L.A., Roberto, G., Grimshaw, J.M., Harvey, E.J., Oxman, A., and Thomson, M.A. (1998). Closing the gap between research and practice: An overview of systematic reviews of interventions to promote the implementation of research findings. *British Medical Journal*, 317(7156): 465–8.

Biehl, J. (2004). The activist state: Global pharmaceuticals, AIDS, and citizenship in Brazil. *Social Text*, 22(3): 105–32.

Binka, F. (2005). Editorial: North–South research collaborations: a move towards a true partnership? *Tropical Medicine and International Health*, 10(3): 207–9.

Black, N. (2001). Evidence based policy: proceed with care. *BMC*, 323: 275–8.

Bloor, D. (1976). *Knowledge and Social Imagery*. London: Routledge.

Bluhm, R. (2005). From hierarchy to network: A richer view of evidence for evidence-based medicine. *Perspectives in Biology and Medicine*, 48(4): 535–48.

Bockting, C.L.H., Boerema, I. and Hermens, M.L.M. (2010). Update multidisciplinaire richtlijn voor de diagnostiek, behandeling en begeleiding van volwassenen met een depressieve stoornis [Update multidisciplinary guideline for the diagnosis, treatment and guidance of adults with a depressive disorder]. *GZ-Psychologie*, 1(1): 40–3.

Bonneuil, C. (2000). Development as experiment: science and state building in late colonial and postcolonial Africa, 1930–1970. *Osiris*, 15: 258–81.

Borders, T.F., Booth, B.M., Han, X., Wright, P., Leukefeld, C., Falck, R.S., et al. (2008). Longitudinal changes in methamphetamine and cocaine use in untreated rural stimulant users: racial differences and the impact of methamphetamine legislation. *Addiction*, 103: 800–8.

Boruch, R.F. (1997). *Randomised Experiments for Planning and Evaluation. A Practical Guide*. London: Sage.

Boyd, K. (2001). Early discontinuation violates Helsinki principles. *BMJ*, 322: 605–6.

Boyer, E.W. and Shannon, M. (2005). The serotonin syndrome. *New England Journal of Medicine*, 352(11): 1112–20.

Brindle, L.A., Oliver, S.E., Dedman, D., Donovan, J.L., Neal, D.E., Hamdy, F.C., Lane, J.A. and Peters, T.J. (2006). Measuring the psychosocial impact of population-based prostate-specific antigen testing for prostate cancer in the UK . *BJU International*, 98(4): 777–82.

Brown, P. and Zavestoski, S. (2005). *Social movements in health.* Oxford: Blackwell Publishing.

Brown, R. (1997a). Artificial experiments on society: Comte, G.C. Lewis and Mill. *Journal of Historical Sociology*, 10(1): 74–97.

Brown, R. (1997b). The delayed birth of social experiments. *History of the Human Sciences*, 10(2): 1–23.

Burns, A., Howard, R., Wilkinson, R.G. and Banerjee, S. (2005). NICE draft guidance on the anti-dementia drugs. *BMJ* [Online]. [Accessed 03 December 2009].

Busfield, J. (2006). Pills, power, people: sociological understandings of the pharmaceutical industry. *Sociology*, 40: 297–314.

Callahan, D. (1987). *Setting Limits: Medical Goals in an Ageing Society*. New York: Simon & Schuster.

Callon, M. (2004). Europe wrestling with technology. *Economy and Society*, 1(33): 121–34.

Callon, M., Lascoumes, P. and Barthe, Y. (2001). *Agir dans un monde uncertain* Paris: Seuil.

Callon, M. and Law, J. (1982). On interests and their transformation: enrolment and counter-enrolment. *Social Studies of Science*, 12: 615–25.

Callon, M. and Rabeharisoa, V. (2008). The growing engagement of emergent concerned groups in political and economic life: lessons from the French Association of Neuromuscular Disease Patients. *Science, Technology & Human Values*, 33(2): 230–61.

Cambrosio, A., Keating, P., Schlich, T. and Weisz, G. (2006). Regulatory objectivity and the generation and management of evidence in medicine. *Social Science & Medicine*, 63: 189–99.

Campbell, M., Fitzpatrick, R., Haines, A., Kinmonth, A.L., Sandercock, P., Spiegelhalter, D. and Tyrer, P. (2000). Framework for design and evaluation of complex interventions to improve health. *British Medical Journal*, 321(7262): 694–6.

Cancer Research UK (2009). Latest UK Cancer Incidence and Mortality Summary – rates. http://info.cancerresearchuk.org/prod_consump/groups/cr_common/@nre/@sta/documents/generalcontent/crukmig_1000ast-2736.pdf. [Accessed February 2010.]

Carrithers, D. (1995). The enlightenment science of society. In: C. Fox, R. Porter and R. Wokler, eds., *Inventing human science. 18th-century domains*, Berkeley, CA: University of California Press, pp. 232–70.

Carroll, K.M. and Onken, L.S. (2005). Behavioral therapies for drug abuse. *American Journal of Psychiatry*, 162(8): 1452–60.

Cartwright, N. (2007). Are RCTs the Gold Standard? *BioSocieties*, 2(1): 11–20.

Chalmers, I. (1990). Underreporting research is scientific misconduct. *JAMA,* 263: 1405–08.

Chalmers, I. (1995). What do I want from health research and researchers when I am a patient? *BMJ*, 310: 1315–8.

Chalmers, I. (2005). Statistical theory was not the reason that randomisation was used in the British Medical Research Council's clinical trial of streptomycin for pulmonary tuberculosis. In: Jorland, G., Opinel, A., Weisz, G., eds. *Body Counts: Medical Quantification in Historical and Sociological Perspectives.* Montreal: McGill-Queens University Press, pp. 309–34.

Chalmers, I. (2007). The Alzheimer's Sciety, drug manufacturers, and public trust. *BMJ*, 335(7616): 40.

Chamberlain, J., Melia, J., Moss, S. and Brown, J. (1997). The diagnosis, management, treatment and costs of prostate cancer in England and Wales. *Health Technology Assessment*, 1 (3) (whole volume).

Chapin, F.S. (1917a). The experimental method and sociology. I. The theory and practice of the experimental method. *Scientific Monthly*, 4 (2): 133–44.

Chapin, F.S. (1917b). The experimental method and sociology. II. Social legislation is social experimentation. *Scientific Monthly*, 4(3): 238–47.

Chapple, A., Ziebland, S., Shepperd, S., Miller, R., Herxheimer, A. and McPherson, A. (2002). Why men with prostate cancer want wider access to prostate specific antigen testing: qualitative study. *British Medical Journal*, 325: 737–41.

Chopra, S.S. (2003). Industry funding of clinical trials: benefit or bias? *JAMA*, 290(1): 113–14.

Collins, H.M. and Pinch, T. (1993). *The Golem: What everyone should know about science*, Cambridge: Cambridge University Press.

Consortium Richtlijnontwikkeling (2009). *Richtlijnherziening van de multidisciplinaire richtlijn depressie bij volwassenen (eerste revisie).* [Consortium Guidelines Development, 2009. *Guideline change of the multidisciplinary guideline depression in adults (first revision).* Utrecht: Trimbos Instituut. Available at www.ggzrichtlijnen.nl/index.php?pagina=/ richtlijn/item/pagina.php&richtlijn_id=88 [accessed 30 March 2010].

Cook, B. and Kothari, U. (eds.) (2001). *Participation – The New Tyranny?* London: Zed Press.

Cook, T.D. and Campbell, D.T. (1979). *Quasi-experimentation. Design and Analysis Issues for Field Settings.* Chicago: Rand McNally.

Cook, R.J. and Sackett, D.L. (1995). The number needed to treat: a clinically useful measure of treatment effect. *BMJ*, 310: 452–4.

Corrigan, O. (2003). Empty ethics: the problem with informed consent. *Sociology of Health and Illness*, 25(7): 768–92.

Coveney, J. (1988). The politics and ethics of health promotion: the importance of Michel Foucault. *Health Education Research*, 13(3): 459–68.

Crinson, I. (2004). The politics of regulation within the 'modernized' NHS: the case of beta interferon and the 'cost-effective' treatment of multiple schlerosis. *Journal of Critical Social Policy*, 24: 30–49.

Culyer, A.J. (1983). Effectiveness and efficiency of health services. *Effective Health Care*, 1: 7–9.

Culyer, A.J. and Meads, A. (1992). The United-Kingdom – effective, efficient, equitable. *Journal of Health Politics, Policy and Law*, 17: 667–88.

Daemmrich, A.A. (2004). *Pharmacopolitics. Drug Regulation in the United States and Germany.* Chapel Hill and London: The University of North Carolina Press.

Danchin, N. (2009). Correspondence: Rosuvastatin, C-reactive protein, LDL cholesterol and the JUPITER trial. *The Lancet*, 374: 24–5.

Danziger, K. (1990). *Constructing the subject.* Cambridge: Cambridge University Press.

Daston, L. and Galison, P. (2007). *Objectivity.* New York: Zone Books.

Dear, P. (2002). Experiment in science and technology studies, in S. Jasanoff (ed), *Science and Technology Studies: International Encyclopedia of Social and Behavioral Sciences.* New York: Elsevier. pp. 277–93.

Dehue, T. (2001). Establishing the experimenting society: The historical origin of social experimentation according to the randomized controlled design. *American Journal of Psychology*, 114(2): 283–302.

Dehue, T. (2002). A Dutch treat. Randomised controlled experimentation and the case of heroin-maintenance in the Netherlands. *History of the Human Sciences*, 15(2): 75–98.

Dehue, T. (2005). History of the control group. In: B. Everitt and D. Howell, eds. *Encyclopedia of Statistics in the Behavioral Sciences*, vol 2. Chichester, UK: Wiley.

Dehue, T. (2008). *De Depressie-epidemie. Over de plicht het lot in eigen hand te nemen* [The Depression-epidemic. On the duty to manage one's destiny]. Amsterdam: Augustus.

Deleuze, G. (2007). Society of Control <http://www.gnn.tv/threads/26172/> [Accessed July 2008].

Department of Health. (2005). *Government Response to NICE Consultation on Alzheimer's Drugs.* London: DoH.

Despres, J.-P. (2009). Bringing JUPITER down to earth. *The Lancet*, 373: 1147–8.

Desrosières, A. (1998). *The Politics of Large Numbers. A History of Statistical Reasoning.* Cambridge, MA: Harvard University Press.

Dickersin, K. (1990). The existence of publication bias and risk factors for its occurrence. *JAMA*, 263(10): 1385–1359.

Dickersin, K., Chan, S., Chalmers, T.C., Sacks, H.S. and Smith, H. (1987). Publication bias and clinical trials. *Controlled Clinical Trials*, 8(4): 343–53.

DIPEX.org – Patient Experiences of Health and Illness. PSA Testing module. <http://www.dipex.org/ psatesting> [accessed July 2008].

Djulbegovic, B., Lacevic, M., Cantor, A., Fields, K.K., Bennett, C.L., Adams, J.R., Kuderer, N.M. and Lyman, G.H. (2000). The uncertainty principle and industry – sponsored research. *The Lancet*, 356: 635–8.

Donovan, J.L., Frankel, S., Faulkner, A., Gillatt, D. and Hamdy, F.C. (1999). Dilemmas in treating early prostate cancer: the evidence and a questionnaire survey of consultant urologists in the UK. *British Medical Journal*, 318: 299–300.

Donovan, J.L., Frankel, S.J., Neal, D.E. and Hamdy, F.C. (2001). Screening for prostate cancer in the UK. *British Medical Journal*, 323: 763–4.

Donovan, J.L., Mills, N., Smith, M., Brindle, L., Jacoby, A., Peters, T., Frankel, S., Neal, D., Hamdy, F. and Little, P. (2002a). Quality improvement report: Improving design and conduct of randomised trials by embedding them in qualitative research: ProtecT (prostate testing for cancer and treatment) study. *British Medical Journal* 325: 766–70.

Donovan, J.L., Brindle, L. and Mills, N. (2002b). Capturing users' experiences of participating in cancer trials. *European Journal of Cancer Care*, 11(3): 210–14.

Donovan, J.L., Hamdy, F., Neal, D., Peters, T., Oliver, S., Brindle, L. et al. (2003). Prostate Testing for Cancer and Treatment (ProtecT) feasibility study. *Health Technology Assessment*, 7, 14 (whole volume).

Doucet, M. and Sismondo, S. (2008). Evaluations of solutions to sponsorship bias. *Journal of Medical Ethics*, 34: 627–30.

Earl-Slater, A. (2002). *The Handbook of Clinical Trials and Other Research*, Oxon: Radcliffe Medical Press.

Eggers, M., Davey-Smith, G. and O'Rourke, T. (2001). The rationale, potentials and promise of systematic reviews, in M. Egger, G. Davey-Smith and D.G. Altman (eds) *Systematic Reviews in Health Care*, London: BMJ.

Elkashef, A., Rawson, R.A., Smith, E., Pearce, V., Flammino, F., Campbell, J., et al. (2007). The NIDA Methamphetamine Clinical Trials Group: a strategy to increase clinical trials research capacity. *Addiction*, 102 Suppl 1: 107–13.

Epstein, S. (1995). The construction of lay expertise: AIDS activism and the forging of credibility in the reform of clinical trials. *Science Technology and Human Values*, 20(4): 408–37.

Epstein, S. (1996). *Impure Science: AIDS, Activism, and the Politics of Knowledge.* Berkeley: University of California Press.

Epstein, S. (1997). Activism, drug regulation, and the politics of therapeutic evaluation in the AIDS era: A case study of ddC and the 'surrogate markers' debate. *Social Studies of Science*, 27(5): 691–726.

Epstein, S. (2007). *Inclusion: The Politics of Difference in Medical Research.* Chicago: University of Chicago Press.

Essink Bot, M.L., de Koning, H.J., Nijs, H.G., Kirkels, W.J., van der Maas, P.J. and Schroder, F.H. (1998). Short-term effects of population based screening for prostate cancer on health-related quality of life. *Journal of the National Cancer Institute*, 90: 925–31.

Evans, R., Edwards, A.G.K., Elwyn, G., Watson, E., Grol, R., Brett, J., Austoker, J. (2007). 'It's a maybe test': men's experiences of prostate specific antigen testing in primary care. *British Journal of General Practice*, 57: 303–10.

Faulkner, A. (1997). 'Strange bedfellows' in the laboratory of the NHS? An analysis of the new science of health technology assessment in the United Kingdom. In:

Elston M.A. (ed.) *The Sociology of Medical Science and Technology.* Sociology of Health and Illness Monograph No. 3, Blackwell: Oxford, pp. 183–207.

Faulkner, A. (2009). *Medical Technology into Healthcare and Society: A Sociology of Devices, Innovation and Governance.* Chapter 5: 'The PSA test for prostate cancer: risk constructs governance?'. Basingstoke: Palgrave Macmillan.

Featherstone, K. and Donovan, J. (1998). Random allocation or allocation at random? Patients' perspectives of participation in a randomised controlled trial. *British Medical Journal*, 317: 1177–80.

Featherstone, K. and Donovan J. (2002) 'Why don't they just tell me straight, why allocate it?' The struggle to make sense of participating in a randomised controlled trial. *Social Science & Medicine*, 55(5): 709–19.

Feeman, W.E. (2009). Correspondence: Rosuvastatin, C-reactive protein, LDL cholesterol and the JUPITER trial. *The Lancet*, 374: 24.

Felt, U., Wynne, B., Callon, M. et al. (2007). *Taking Knowledge Society Seriously: Report of the Expert group on Science and Governance.* Brussels: Science, Economy and Society Directorate, European Commission.

Ferguson, N. (2004). *Osteoporosis in focus.* London: Pharmaceutical Press.

Fisher, J.A. (2009). *Medical Reseach for Hire.* New Brunswick, NJ: Rutgers University Press.

Fishman, J.R. (2004). Manufacturing Desire: The Commodification of Female Sexual Dysfunction. *Social Studies of Science*, 34(2): 187–218.

Folstein, M.F., Folstein, S.E. and McHugh, P.R. (1975). Mini – Mental State – Practical Method for Grading Cognitive State of Patients for Clinician. *Journal of Psychiatric Research*, 12: 189–98.

Food and Drug Administration. (1981). The story of the laws behind the labels. Available at www.fda.gov/AboutFDA/WhatWeDo/History/Overviews/ucm056044.htm [accessed 8 March 2010].

Foucault, M. (1979). Pastoral Power and Political Reason, in Carrette, J.R. (ed.) (1999). *Religion and Culture*, Manchester: Manchester University Press, pp. 135–53.

Foucault, M. (1980). The eye of power. In: Gordon, C. (ed.). *Power/Knowledge: Selected Interviews and Other Writings 1972–77.* New York, Pantheon Books, pp. 146–65.

Fournier, J.C. (2010). Antidepressant drug effects and depression severity. A patient-level meta-analysis. *Journal of the American Medical Association*, 303 (1): 47–53.

Fox, R.C. (1957). Training for Uncertainty. In: R.K. Merton, G. Reader and P.L. Kendall (eds), *The Student Physician.* Cambridge: Harvard University Press, pp. 207–41.

Fox, R.C. (1959). *Experiment Perilous: Physicians and Patients Facing the Unknown.* New York: The Free Press.

Fox, R.C. (1980). The Evolution of Medical Uncertainty. *Milbank Memorial Fund Quarterly*, 58(1): 1–49.

Fox, R.C. (2000). Medical Uncertainty Revisited. In: G. L. Albrecht, R. Fitzpatrick and S.C. Scrimshaw (eds), *The Handbook of Social Studies in Health and Medicine* London: SAGE Publications, pp. 409–25.

Franklin, S. (2003). Ethical Biocapital: New Strategies of Cell Culture. In: S. Franklin and M. Lock (eds), *Remaking Life and Death: Toward an Anthropology of the Biosciences*. Santa Fe, NM: School of American Research Press, pp. 97–128.

Fraser (MP). (2006). House of Commons Written Answers for 14 Dec 2006 – Cancer Treatment. http://www.parliament.the-stationery-office.com/pa/cm200607/cmhansrd/cm061218/text/61218w0061.htm. [Accessed March 2010].

Freidson, E. (1984). The changing nature of professional control. *Annual Review of Sociology*, 10: 1–20.

Freidson, E. (1988). *Profession of Medicine: A Study of the Sociology of Applied Knowledge*. Chicago: University of Chicago Press.

Friedli, L. (2009). *Mental Health, Resilience and Inequalities*. WHO Europe, available at www.euro.who.int/document/e92227.pdf [accessed on 30 March 2010].

Fullerton, H.R. and Bishop, E.L. (1933). Improved rural housing as a factor in malaria control. *South. Medical Journal*, 26: 465–8.

Galton, F. (1872). Statistical inquiries into the efficacy of prayer. *Fortnightly Review* 12: 124–35.

Galton, F. (1889). Human variety. *Journal of the Anthropological Institute*, 18: 401–19.

Garcia de Tena, J. (2009). Rosuvastatin, C-reactive protein, LDL cholesterol and the JUPITER trial. *The Lancet*, 374: 24.

Garratini, S. and Chalmers, I. (2009). Patients and the public deserve big changes in the evaluation of drugs. *British Medical Journal*, 338: 804–6.

Geissler, P.W. and Pool, R. (2006). Popular concerns with medical research projects in Africa – a critical voice in debates about overseas research ethics. *Tropical Medicine and International Health*, 11(7): 975–82.

Geissler, P.W., Kelly, A., Imokhuede, B. and Pool, R. (2008) 'He is now like a brother, I can even give him my blood' – relational ethics and material exchanges in a malaria vaccine 'trial community' in The Gambia. *Social Science and Medicine*, 67(5): 696–709.

Gezondheidsraad (2006). *Verzekeringsgeneeskundige protocollen. Algemene inleiding, overspanning, depressieve stoornis* [Health Council, 2006. Health Insurance protocols. General introduction, stress, depressive disorder]. Den Haag: Gezondheidsraad, available at www.gezondheidsraad.nl/sites/default/files/200622_site3.pdf [accessed 30 March 2010].

Gibbons, M. (1999). Science's New Social Contract with Society. *Nature* 402: C81–84.

Gibbons, M., Limoges, C., Schwartzman, S., Nowotny, H., Trow, M. and Scott, P. (1994). *The New Production of Knowledge: The Dynamics of Science and Research in Contemporary Societies.* Newbury Park, CA.: Sage.

Giddens, A. (1991). *The Consequences of Modernity*, Stanford, CA: Stanford University Press.

Gimming, J.E. and Slutsker, L. (2009). House screening for malaria control. *The Lancet*, 374: 945–55.

Godwin, M., Ruhland, L., Casson, I., MacDonald, S., Delva, D., Birtwhistle, R., Lam, M. and Seguin, R. (2003). Pragmatic controlled clinical trials in primary care: the struggle between external and internal validity. *BMC Medical Research Methodology* 3: 28.

Goffman, E. (1959). *The Presentation of Self in Everyday Life.* New York: The Overlook Press.

Graf, C., Battisti, W.P., Bridges, D., Bruce-Winkler, V., Conaty, J.M., Ellison, J.M., Field, E.A., Gurr, J.A., Marx, M-E., Patel, M., Sanes-Miller, C., Yarker, Y.E. for the International Society for Medical Publication Professionals (2009). Good publication practice for communicating company sponsored medical research: the GPP2 Guidlelines. *British Medical Journal* 339: b4330.

Grant, C.H.I., Cissna, K.N. et al. (2000). Patients' perceptions of physicians communication and outcomes of the accrual to trial process. *Health Communication*, 12(1): 23–39.

Gray, A., and S. Harrison, eds. (2004). *Governing Medicine: Theory and Practice.* Maidenhead and New York: Open University Press.

Greenhalgh,T. (1997). How to read a paper: papers that report drug trials, *British Medical Journal*, 315: 480–83.

Grol, R. and Grimshaw, J. (2003). From best evidence to best practice: effective implementation of change in patients' care. *The Lancet*, 362: 1225–30.

Grossman, J. and MacKenzie, F.J. (2005). The randomized controlled trial: gold standard or merely standard. *Perspectives in Biology and Medicine*, 48(4): 516–34.

Guyatt, G.H., Sackett, D.L. and Cook, D.J. (1993). Users' guides to the medical literature. II. How to use an article about therapy or prevention. *Journal of the American Medical Association*, 270 (21): 2598–601.

Hacking, I. (1990). *The Taming of Chance.* New York: Cambridge University Press.

Halpern, S.A. (2004). *Lesser Harms: The Morality of Risk in Medical Research.* Chicago: University of Chicago Press.

Ham, C. and Roberts, G. (eds) (2003). *Reasonable Rationing: International Experience of Priority Setting in Health Care.* Maidenhead: Open University Press.

Hayden, C. (2003). *When Nature Goes Public: The Making and Unmaking of Bioprospecting in Mexico.* Princeton: Princeton University Press.

Hayden, C. (2007). Taking as Giving. *Social Studies of Science*, 37(5): 729–58.

Healy, D. (1997). *The Antidepressant Era.* Cambridge: Harvard University Press.

Healy, D. (2004). *Let Them Eat Prozac: The Unhealthy Relationship Between the Pharmaceutical Industry and Depression.* New York: New York University Press.

Healy, D. (2009). Trussed in evidence? Ambiguities at the interface between clinical evidence and clinical practice. *Transcultural Psychiatry,* 46(1): 16–37.

Heimer, C.A. (2007). Old inequalities, new diseases: HIV/AIDS in Sub-Saharan Africa. *Annual Review of Sociology,* 33: 551–77.

Helms, R. (2002). *Guinea Pig Zero. An Anthology of the Journal for Human Research Subjects.* New Orleans: Garrett County Press.

Hewitson, P. and Austoker, J. (2005). Part 2: Patient information, informed decision-making and the psycho-social impact of prostate-specific antigen testing. *BJU International,* 95(S3): 16–32.

Hlatky, M.A. (2008). Expanding the orbit of primary prevention – moving beyond JUPITER, *New England Journal of Medicine,* 359(21): 2280–82.

Holmes D.R. and Marcus G.E. (2005). Cultures of expertise and the management of globalisation: toward the re-functioning of ethnography. In: Ong, A. and Collier S.J. (eds) *Global Assemblages: Technology, Politics and Ethics as Anthropological Problems.* Oxford: Blackwell Publishing. pp. 236–52.

Holton, G. (1978). Subelectrons, presuppositions, and the Millikan-Ehrenhaft dispute. *Historical Studies in the Physical Sciences,* 9: 161–224.

Horton, R. (1995). The rhetoric of research. *British Medical Journal,* 310: 985–7.

Horton, R. (1997). Conflicts of interest in clinical research: opprobium or obsession? *The Lancet,* 349: 1112–1113.

Horton, R. (2002). Postpublication criticism and the shaping of clinical knowledge. *Journal of the American Medical Association,* 287: 2843–7.

Horton, R. (2003a). Statin wars: why Astra Zeneca must retreat. *The Lancet,* 362: 1341.

Horton, R. (2003b). Editor's reply. *The Lancet,* 362: 1856.

Ioannidis, J.P.A. (2008). Effectiveness of antidepressants: an evidence myth constructed from a thousand randomized trials? *Philosophy, Ethics, and Humanities in Medicine,* 3 (14). Available at www.peh-med.com/content/pdf/1747-5341-3-14.pdf [accessed 30 March 2010].

Irving, P. (2005). Anger at drugs removal. *The Times,* 10 March 2005.

Irwin, A. and Michael, M. (2003). *Science, social theory and public knowledge* Milton Keynes: Open University Press.

Jarvis, M. (2004). *Psychodynamic Psychology: Classical Theory and Contemporary Research.* London: Thomson.

Jasanoff, S. (2005). *Designs on Nature: Science and Democracy in Europe and the United States.* Princeton: Princeton University Press.

Jenkins, V., Fallowfield, L.J., Souhami, R.L., Sawtell, M. (1999). How do doctors explain randomised clinical trials to their patients? *European Journal of Cancer,* 35: 1187–93.

Jonvallen, P. (2005). *Testing Pills, Enacting Obesity: The Work of Localizing Tools in a Clinical Trial.* Department of Technology and Social Change. Linköping, Linköping University. Unpublished PhD thesis.

Kachur, S.P., Abdulla S., Barnes K., Mshinda H., Durrehim, D., Kitua, A., Bloland, P. (2001) Complex and large trials of pragmatic malaria interventions. *Tropical Medicine International Health*, 6: 324–5.

Kaptchuck, T. (2001). The double-blind, randomised, placebo-controlled trial: Gold standard or golden calf? *Journal of Clinical Epidemiology*, 54(6): 541–9.

Katz, J. (2002). From how to why: on luminous description and causal inference in ethnography (part 2). *Ethnography*, 3: 63–90.

Keating, P. and Cambrosio, A. (2003). *Biomedical platforms. realigning the normal and the pathological in late-twentieth-century medicine.* Cambridge, MA: MIT Press.

Keating, P. and Cambrosio, A. (2005). Risk on trial: the interaction of innovation and risk factors in clinical trials. In: T. Schlich and U. Throhler (eds), *The Risks of Medical Innovation: Risk Perception and Assessment in Historical Context,* London: Routledge. pp. 225–41.

Keating, P. and Cambrosio, A. (2007). Cancer clinical trials: The emergence and development of a new style of practice. *Bulletin of the History of Medicine*, 81(1): 197–223.

Kelly, A. (in press). Pragmatic clinical research: remember Bambali: evidence, ethics and the co-production of truth. In: P.W. Geissler and C. Molyneux (eds) *Ethics and Ethnography.* Oxford: Berghahn.

Kernick, D.P. (2003). Correspondence: Statin Wars. *The Lancet*, 362: 1855.

Killeen, G.F. (2003). Following in Soper's footsteps: northeast Brazil 63 years after eradication of Anopheles gambiae. *Lancet Infectious Disease*, 3: 663–6.

Kimmelman, J. (2007). The therapeutic misconception at 25: treatment, research and confusion. *Hastings Center Report*, 37(6): 36–42.

Kirby M., Ameh, D., Bottomley, C., Green, C. Jawara, M., Milligan P.J., Snell, P., Conway, D., Lindsay, S.W. (2009). Effect of two different house screening interventions on exposure to malaria vectors and on anaemia in children in The Gambia: a randomised controlled trial. *The Lancet*, 374: 998–1009.

Kirsch, I., et al. (2008). Initial severity and antidepressant benefits: A meta analysis of data submitted to the Food and Drug Administration. *PloS Medicine*, 5(2): 260–8. Available at www.plosmedicine.org/article/info:doi/10.1371/journal. pmed.0050045 [accessed 8 March 2010].

Knorr Cetina, K. (1999). *Epistemic Cultures. How the Sciences make Knowledge.* Cambridge, MA and London, UK: Harvard University Press.

Kritiek P. and Campion E.W. (2009). JUPITER Clinical Directions – polling results, *NEJM*, 360: 10.

Kuhn, T.S. (1962). *The Structure of Scientific Revolutions.* Chicago: University of Chicago Press.

Kurer, O. (1991). *John Stuart Mill. The Politics of Progress.* New York: Garland.

Lagakos, S.W. (2006). The challenge of subgroup analyses – reporting without distorting. *New England Journal of Medicine*, 354: 1667–9.

Lairumbi, G.M., Molyneux, S., Snow, R.W., Marsh, K., Peshu, N., English, M. (2008). Promoting the social value of research in Kenya: Examining the practical aspects of collaborative partnerships using an ethical framework. *Social Science & Medicine*, 67(5): 734–47.

Lakoff, A. (2005). *Pharmaceutical Reason: Knowledge and Value in Global Psychiatry.* Cambridge: Cambridge University Press.

Lakoff, A. (2007). The right patients for the drug: managing the placebo effect in antidepressant trials. *BioSocieties*, 2(1): 57–71.

Landelijke Stuurgroep multidisciplinaire richtlijnontwikkeling, 2005a. Multidisciplinaire richtlijnen schizofrenie en depressie gereed. Een feestelijke presentatie [National Steering Committe Development Multidisciplinary Guidelines, 2005a. Multidisciplinary guidelines schizofrenia and depression finished. A festive presentation]. Nieuwsbrief GGZ-R, 4, (7). Available at www.ggzrichtlijnen.nl/uploaded/docs/Nieuwsbrief GGZ-R no. 7.pdf [accessed 8 March 2010].

Landelijke Stuurgroep Multidisciplinaire Richtlijnontwikkeling, 2005b. Multidisciplinaire richtlijn depressie [National Steering Committe Development Multidisciplinary Guidelines, 2005b. Multidisciplinary guideline depression]. Utrecht: Trimbos Instituut. Available at www.ggzrichtlijnen.nl/uploaded/docs/AF0605SAMENVRichtlDepressie.pdf [accessed 8 March 2010].

Langley, C., Gray, S., Selley, S., Bowie, C., Price, C. (2000). Clinicians' attitudes to recruitment to randomised trials in cancer care: a qualitative study. *Journal of Health Services Research Policy*, 5(3): 164–9.

Latour, B. (1987). *Science in Action,* Cambridge MA: Harvard University Press.

Latour, B. (1993). *We Have Never Been Modern.* Cambridge, MA: Harvard University Press.

Latour, B. (1998). From the world of science to the world of research? *Science*, 280: 208–09.

Latour, B. (2004). *Politics of Nature: How to Bring the Sciences into Democracy.* Harvard: Harvard University Press.

Latour, B. and Woolgar, S. (1979). *Laboratory Life: The Construction of Scientific Facts.* Princeton, NJ: Princeton University Press.

Leach, M., Fairhead, J. and Small, M. (2004). *Childhood Vaccination and Society in the Gambia: Public Engagement with Science and Delivery.* IDS Working Papers. Brighton: University of Sussex.

Leach, M., Scones, I. and Wynne, B. (eds), (2005). *Science and Citizenship*, London: Zed Press.

Leahey, E. (2008). Overseeing research practice: the case of data editing. *Science, Technology and Human Values*, 33: 605–30.

Leichsenring, F. (2005). Are psychoanalytic and psychodynamic psychotherapies effective? A review. *International Journal of Psychoanalysis*, 86(3): 841–68.

Lewis, C.G. (1852, reprint 1974). *A Treatise on the Methods of Observation and Reasoning in Politics.* Vol. 1. New York: Arno Press.

Lezaun, J. and Soneryd, L. (2007). Consulting citizens: technologies of elicitation and the mobility of publics. *Public Understanding of Science*, 16: 279–97.

Lidz, C.W., Appelbaum, P.S., Grisso, T. and Renaud, M. (2004). Therapeutic misconception and the appreciation of risks in clinical trials. *Social Science and Medicine*, 58(9): 1689–97.

Light, D.W. (1991). Professionalism as a countervailing power. *Journal of Health Politics, Policy and Law*, 16: 499–506.

Light, D. and Levine, S. (1988). The changing character of the medical-profession – a theoretical overview. *Milbank Quarterly*, 66: 10–32.

Light, D.W. and Hughes, D. (2001). Introduction: A sociological perspective on rationing: power, rhetoric and situated practices. *Sociology of Health & Illness*, 23: 551–69.

Lindegger, G., Milford, C., Slack, C., Quayle, M., Xaba, X. and Vardas, E. (2006). Beyond the checklist: assessing understanding for HIV vaccine trial participation in South Africa. *Journal of Acquired Immune Deficiency Syndrome*, 43(5): 560–66.

Lindsay, S.W., Jawara, M., Paine, K., Pinder, M., Walraven, G.E.L., Emerson, P.M. (2003). Changes in house design reduce exposure to malaria mosquitoes. *International Journal of Tropical Health*, 8: 512–17.

Loveman, E., Green, C., Kirkby, J., Takeda, A., Picot, J., Bradbury, J., Payne, E. and Clegg, A. (2005). The clinical and cost-effectiveness of donepezil, rivastigmine, galantamine, and memantine for Alzheimer's disease. Southhampton: Southampton Health Technology Assessment Centre.

Lovie, A.D. (1979). The analysis of variance in experimental psychology: 1934–1945. *British Journal of Mathematical and Statistical Psychology*, 32(2): 151–78.

Lurie P. and Wolfe, S.M. (1997). Unethical trials of interventions to reduce perinatal transmission of the human immunodeficiency virus in developing countries. *New England Journal of Medicine*, 337: 847–9.

Macklin, R. (2004). Double standards in medical research in developing countries. *Cambridge Law and Ethics Series*, No. 2. Cambridge: Cambridge University Press.

Maeseneer, J.M.D., Van Driel, M.L., Gren, L.A. and Van Weel, C. (2003). The need for research in primary care. *The Lancet*, 362: 1314–19.

Marks, H.M. (1997). *The Progress of Experiment. Science and Therapeutic Reform in the United States, 1900–1990.* New York: Cambridge University Press.

Marks, H.M. (2000). Trust and mistrust in the marketplace: statistics and clinical research, 1945–1960. *History of Science*, 38: 343–55.

Marres, N. (2007). The issues deserve more credit: Pragmatist contributions to the study of public involvement in controversy. *Social Studies of Science*, 37(5): 759–80.

Marres, N. (2009). Testing powers of engagement: green living experiments, the ontological turn and the undoability of involvement. *European Journal of Social Theory*, 12(1): 117–33.

May, C. (2006). Mobilizing modern facts: Health Technology Assessment and the politics of evidence. *Sociology of Health & Illness*, 28: 513–32.

May, C. and Ellis, N.T. (2001). When protocols fail: technical evaluation, biomedical knowledge, and the social production of 'facts' about a telemedicine clinic. *Social Science and Medicine*, 53: 989–1002.

McCall, W.A. (1923). *How to Experiment in Education*. New York: Macmillan.

McDonald, R. (2002). Street-level bureaucrats? Heart disease, health economics and policy in a primary care group. *Health Social Care Community*, 10: 129–35.

McDonald, A.M., Knight, R.C., Campbell, M.K., Entwistle, V.A., Grant, A.M., Cook, J.A. (2006). What influences recruitment to randomised controlled trials? A review of trials funded by two UK funding agencies. *Trials*, 7:9 online doi:10.1186/1745-6215-7-9.

McGoey, L. (2007). On the will to ignorance in bureaucracy. *Economy and Society* 36: 212–35.

McGoey, L. (2009). Pharmaceutical controversies and the performative value of uncertainty, *Science as Culture* 18(2): 151–67.

McGoey, L. (2010). Profitable failure: antidepressant drugs and the triumph of flawed experiments. *History of the Human Sciences*, 23(1): 58–78.

McGuire, A., Henderson, G., Mooney, G. (1986). *The Economics of Health Care: An Introductory Text*. London: Routledge.

McPherson, K. (1994). The best and the enemy of the good: randomised controlled trials, uncertainty, and assessing the role of patient choice in medical decision making. *Journal of Epidemiology and Community Health*, 48: 6–15.

Mechanic, D. (1995). Dilemmas in rationing health care services: the case for implicit rationing, *British Medical Journal*, 310: 1655–9.

Medawar, C. et al. (2002). Paroxetine, panorama and user reporting of ADRs: Consumer intelligence matters in clinical practice and post-marketing drug surveillance. *International Journal of Risk & Safety in Medicine*, 15: 161–169. Available at www.socialaudit.org.uk/ijrsm-161-169.pdf [accessed 9 March 2010].

Medical Research Council PR06 collaborators (2004). Early closure of a randomised controlled trial of three treatment approaches to early localised prostate cancer: the MRC PR06 trial. *BJU International*, 94(9): 1400–1.

Milewa, T. (2006). Health technology adoption and the politics of governance in the UK. *Social Science & Medicine*, 63: 3102–12.

Mill, J.S. (1843, reprint 1973). *A System of Logic*. Toronto: University of Toronto Press.

Miller, D. (2003). The Virtual Moment. *Journal of the Royal Anthropological Institute*, 9(1): 57–5.

Miller, F.G. and Rosentstein, D.L. (2003). The therapeutic orientation to clinical trials. *New England Journal of Medicine*, 348(14): 1383–6.

Mills, N., Donovan, J.L., Smith, M., Jacoby, A., Neal, D.E., Hamdy, F.C. (2003). Perceptions of equipoise are crucial to trial participation: a qualitative study of men in the ProtecT study. *Controlled Clinical Trials*, 24(3): 272–82.

Mirowski, P., and Van Horn, R. (2005). The contract research organization and the commercialization of scientific research. *Social Studies of Science*, 35(4): 506–48.

Moerman, D.E. (2002). *Meaning, Medicine and the 'Placebo effect'*. Cambridge: Cambridge University Press.

Mol, A. (2008). *The Logic of Care. Health and the Problem of Patient Choice*. London: Routledge.

Molyneux, S. and Geissler, P.W. (2008). Ethics and the ethnography of medical research in Africa. *Social Science & Medicine*, 67(5): 685–95.

Moreira, T. (2005). Diversity in clinical guidelines: the role of repertoires of evaluation. *Social Science and Medicine*, 60(9): 1975–85.

Moreira, T. (2006). Sleep, health and the dynamics of biomedicine. *Social Science & Medicine*, 63(1): 54–63.

Moreira, T. (2007). Entangled evidence: knowledge making in systematic reviews in healthcare. *Sociology of Health & Illness*, 29(2): 180–97.

Moreira, T. (2008). Continuous positive airway pressure machines and the work of coordinating technologies at home. *Chronic Illness*, 4(2): 102–9.

Moreira, T. (2009). Testing promises: truth and hope in drug development and evaluation in Alzheimer's Disease. In: Ballenger, J.F., Whitehouse, P.J., Lyketsos, C., Rabins, P. and Karlawish, J.H.T. (eds) *Do we Have a Pill for That? Interdisciplinary Perspectives on the Development, Use and Evaluation of Drugs in the Treatment of Dementia*. Baltimore: Johns Hopkins University Press.

Moreira, T., May, C. and Bond, J. (2009). Regulatory objectivity in action: MCI and the collective production of uncertainty. *Social Studies of Science*, 39(5): 665–90.

Moreira, T. and Palladino, P. (2005). Between truth and hope: on Parkinson's disease, neurotransplantation and the production of the 'self'. *History of the Human Sciences*, 18(3): 55–82.

National Institute of Clinical Excellence (2001). *Donepezil, Rivastigmine, Galantamine for the Treatment of Alzheimer's Disease*. London: NICE.

National Institute of Health and Clinical Excellence (2002). *Guidance on Cancer Services. Improving Outcomes in Urological Cancers. The Manual*. London: National Institute for Health & Clinical Excellence. <http://www.nice.org.uk/> [Accessed September 2007.]

National Institute of Health and Clinical Excellence (2006). *Appraisal Consultation Document: Donepezil, Rivastigmine, Galantamine and Memantine for the Treatment of Alzheimer's Disease*. London: NICE.

Naylor, C.D., Chen, E. and Strauss, B. (1996). Measured enthusiasm: does the method of reporting trial results alter perceptions of therapeutic effectiveness? *Annals of Internal Medicine*, 117: 916–21.

Norheim, O.F. (2002). The role of evidence in health policy making: a normative perspective. *Health Care Analysis*, 10: 309–17.

Nowotny, H., Scott, P., Gibbons, M. (2001). *Re-thinking Science: Knowledge and the Public in an Age of Uncertainty*. Cambridge: Polity Press.

Oliver, S.E., May, M.T. and Gunnell, D. (2001). International trends in prostate-cancer mortality in the 'PSA ERA'. *International Journal of Cancer*, 92: 893–8.

Oliver, S.E., Donovan, J.L., Peters T.J., Frankel, S., Hamdy, F.C. and Neal, D.E. (2003). Recent trends in the use of radical prostatectomy in England: the epidemiology of diffusion. *BJU International*, 91(4): 331–6.

Orenstein, A.J. (1912). Screening as an antimalaria measure. A contribution to the study of the value of screened dwellings in malaria regions. *Proceedings of Canal Zone Medical Association*, 5:12–18.

Orr, J. (2006). *Panic Diaries: A Genealogy of Panic Disorder*. Durham: Duke University Press.

Orr, L.L. (1999). *Social Experiments. Evaluating Public Programs with Experimental Methods*. London: Sage.

Oudshoorn, N. (1993). United we stand – the pharmaceutical industry, laboratory and clinic in the development of sex-hormones into scientific drugs, 1920–1940. *Science, Technology and Human Values*, 18(1): 5–24.

Parker, G., Anderson, I.M. and Haddad, P. (2001). Clinical trials of antidepressant medications are producing meaningless results. *British Journal of Psychiatry*, 183: 102–04.

Parsons, T. (1951). *The Social System*. Glencoe, IL: The Free Press.

Petryna, A. (2002). *Life Exposed: Biological Citizens after Chernobyl*. Princeton: Princeton University Press.

Petryna, A. (2007). Clinical Trials Offshored: On Private Sector Science and Public Health. *Biosocieties*, 2(1): 21–40.

Petryna, A. (2009). *When Experiments Travel: Clinical Trials and the Global Search for Human Subjects*. Princeton, NJ: Princeton University Press.

Petryna, A. and Kleinman, A. (2006). The pharmaceutical nexus: an introduction. In: A. Petryna, A. Lakoff, and A. Kleinman (eds) *Global Pharmaceuticals: Ethics, Markets, Practices*. Durham, NC: Duke University Press.

PloS Medicine editors. (2009). Ghostwriting: the dirty little secret of medicine that just got bigger. *PloS Medicine*, 6(9): 1–2 Available at www.plosmedicine.org/article/info%3Adoi%2F10.1371%2Fjournal.pmed.1000156 [accessed 8 March 2010].

Porter, T.M. (1986). *The Rise of Statistical Thinking, 1820–1900*. Princeton: Princeton University Press.

Porter, T.M. (1995). *Trust in Numbers. The Pursuit of Objectivity in Science and Public Life*. Princeton: Princeton University Press.

Public Accounts Committee (2005). *Cancer – The Patient's Experience*. PAC Publications. Uncorrected Evidence, House of Commons HC 485-i.

Rabeharisoa, V. and Callon, M. (2002). The involvement of patients' associations in research. *International Social Science Journal*, 54(1): 57.

Radley, D.C., Finkelstein, S.N. and Stafford, R.S. (2006). Off-label prescribing among office-based physicians. *Archives of Internal Medicine*, 166(9): 1021–26.

Rajan, K.S. (2002). Biocapital as an emergent form of life: speculations on the figure of the experimental subject. In: Novas, C. and Gibbons, S. (eds) *Biosocialities, Genetics and The Social Sciences*. London: Routledge.

Rajan, K.S. (2003). Genomic capital: public cultures and markets logics of corporate biotechnology. *Science as Culture*, 12(1): 87–121.

Rajan, K.S. (2006). *Biocapital: The Constitution of Postgenomic Life*. Durham CA: Duke University Press.

Rapley, T., May, C. et al. (2006). Doctor-patient interaction in a randomised controlled trial of decision-support tools. *Social Science & Medicine* 62(9): 2267–78.

Rasmussen, N. (2004). The moral economy of the drug company-medical scientist collaboration in interwar America. *Social Studies of Science*, 34: 161–86.

Rasmussen, N. (2005). The drug industry and clinical research in interwar America: three types of physician collaborator. *Bulletin of the History of Medicine*, 79: 50–80.

Rawlins, M.D. and Culyer, A.J. (2004). National Institute for Clinical Excellence and its value judgments. *British Medical Journal*, 329: 224–7.

Richards, E. (1991). *Vitamin C and Cancer: Medicine or Politics?* New York: St Martin's Press.

Ridker, P.M., Danielson, E., Fonseca, F.A.H., et al., on behalf of the JUPITER Trial Study Group. (2009). Reduction in C-reactive protein and LDL cholesterol and cardiovascular event rates after initiation of rosuvastatin: a prospective study of the JUPITER trial, *The Lancet*, 373: 1175–82.

Rip, A. (1986). Controversies as informal technology-assessment. *Knowledge-Creation Diffusion Utilization*, 8: 349–71.

Roll, J.M. (2007). Contingency management: an evidence-based component of methamphetamine use disorder treatments. *Addiction*, 102(Suppl. 1): 114–40.

Rose, D. & Blume, S. (2003). Citizens as users of technology: an exploratory study of vaccines and vaccination. In: Oudshoorn, N., Pinch, T. (eds). *How Users Matter: The Co-construction of Users and Technology*. Cambridge, MA: MIT Press, pp. 103–31.

Rosenberg, C.E. (2002). The tyranny of diagnosis. Specific entities and individual experience. *The Milbank Quarterly*, 80(2): 237–60.

Rosenberg, C.E. (2003). What is a disease? *Bulletin of the History of Medicine*, 77(3): 491–505.

Rosenstein, R. and Parra, D. (2009). Correspondence: Rosuvastatin, C-reactive protein, LDL cholesterol and the JUPITER trial. *The Lancet*, 374: 24.

Royal College of Psychiatry. (2006). *Implementation of the NICE Guidance on Donepezil, Galantamine, Rivastigmine and Memantine for the Treatment of Alzheimer's Sisease*. London: RCP.

Rucci, A.J. and Tweney, R.D. (1980). Analysis of variance and the 'second discipline' of scientific psychology: A historical account. *Psychological bulletin*, 87: 166–84.

Ryan, S., Williams, I. and Mciver, S. (2007). Seeing the NICE side of cost effectiveness analysis: a qualitative investigation of the use of CEA in NICE technology appraisals. *Health Economics*, 16: 179–93.

Sackett, D.L. (1979). Bias in analytic research. *Journal of Chronic Disease,* 32(1–2): 51–63.

Sackett, D., Straus, S.E., Richardson, W.S., Rosenberg, W. and Haynes, R.B. (2000). *Evidence-based Medicine*. London: Churchill Livingstone.

SAMHSA. (2007). *Results from the 2006 National Survey on Drug Use and Health: National Findings.* Rockville, MD: Office of Applied Studies.

Sana, M. and Weinreb, A. (2008) Insiders, outsiders, and the editing of inconsistent survey data. *Sociological Methods & Research*, 36: 515.

Savage P., Bates C., Abel P. and Waxman, J. (1997). British urological surgery practice: 1. Prostate cancer. *British Journal of Urology*, 79(5): 749–54.

Schaffer, S. (2005). Sky, heaven and the seat of power. In: B. Latour and P. Weibel (eds), *Making Things Public*. Karlsruhe and Cambridge MA: ZKM/MIT Press. pp. 120–25.

Schofield, C.J. and White, G.B. (1984). Engineering against insect-borne diseases in the domestic environment. House design and domestic vectors of disease. *Transactions of Royal Society Tropical Medicine Hygiene*, 78: 285–92.

Schröder, F., Hugosson, J., Roobol, M.J., and 20 others. (2009). Screening and prostate-cancer mortality in a randomized European study. *New England Journal of Medicine*, 360(13): 1320–28.

Selley, S., Donovan, J., Faulkner, A., Coast, J., Gillatt, D. (1997). Diagnosis, management and screening of early localised prostate cancer. *Health Technology Assessment*, 1(2): 1–96 (whole volume).

Shapin, S. and Schaffer, S. (1985). *Leviathan and the Air-Pump. Hobbes, Boyle and Experimental Life*, Princeton: Princeton University Press.

Shuchman, M. (2007). Commercializing clinical trials: risks and benefits of the CRO boom. *New England Journal of Medicine*, 357(14): 1365–68.

Simes, R.J. (1986). Publication bias: the case for an international registry of clinical trials. *Journal of Clinical Oncology*, 4(10): 1529–41.

Sismondo, S. (2007). Ghost management: How much of the medical literature is shaped behind the scenes by the pharmaceutical industry? *PLoS Medicine*, 4(9): e286.

Sismondo, S. (2008). How pharmaceutical industry funding affects trial outcomes: causal structures and responses. *Social Science & Medicine*, 66: 1909–14.

Sismondo, S. (2009). Ghosts in the machine. Publication planning in the medical sciences. *Social Studies of Science*, 39: 171–98.

Smith, R. (1991). Where is the wisdom? The poverty of medical evidence. *British Medical Journal*, 303(6806): 798–9.

Snedecor, G.W. (1936). The improvement of statistical techniques in biology. *Journal of the American Statistical Association*, 31: 690–701.

Sniderman, A.D. (2009). Correspondence: Rosuvastatin, C-reactive protein, LDL cholesterol and the JUPITER trial. *The Lancet*, 374: 24.

Star, S.L. (1991). Invisible work and silenced dialogues in knowledge representation. In: Eriksson, I. V., Kitchenham, B.A. and Tijdens, K.G. (eds) *Women, work and computerization: Understanding and overcoming bias in work and education.* Amsterdam: North-Holland.

Star, S.L. (1991). Power, technologies and the phenomenology of conventions: on being allergic to onions. In Law, J. (ed.). *A Sociology of Monsters: Essays on Power, Technology and Domination.* London: Routledge.

Stengers, I. (2000). *The Invention of Modern Science*, Minneapolis/London: University of Minnesota Press.

Strathern, M. (2000). Accountability … and ethnography. In: M. Strathern (ed.), *Audit Cultures: Anthropological Studies in Accountability, Ethics, and the Academy*, London: Routledge, pp. 279–304.

Strathern, M. (2002). Externalities in comparative guise. *Economy and Society*, 31: 205–67.

Strathern, M. (2004 [1991]). *Partial Connections*. Updated edition. Walnut Creek: Altamira Press.

Strauss, A.L. (1993). *Continual Permutations of Action.* New York: Walter de Gruyter, Inc.

Street, Alice. n.d. Research in the clinic: scientific emplacement and medical failure, Conference Paper *Publics of Public Health*, Kilifi, Kenya, December 7th–11th 2009.

Tanenbaum, S.J. (1994). Knowing and acting in medical research: the epistemological politics of outcomes research. *Journal of Health Politics, Policy and Law*, 19: 27–44.

The Lancet (2006). Rationing is essential in tax-funded health systems. *The Lancet*, 368: 1394.

Thornton, H. (2008). Patient and public involvement in clinical trials. *British Medical Journal*, 336: 903–04.

Timmermans, S. and Alison, A. (2001). Evidence-based medicine, clinical uncertainty, and learning to doctor. *Journal of Health and Social Behavior*, 42(4): 342–59.

Timmermans, S. and Berg, M. (2003). *The Gold Standard: The Challenge of Evidence-based Medicine and Standardization in Health Care.* Philadelphia, PA: Temple University Press.

Timmermans, S. and McKay, T. (2009). Clinical trials as treatment option: bioethics and health care disparities in substance dependency. *Social Science & Medicine*, 69(12): 1784–90.

Timmermans, S. and Tavory, I. (2007). Advancing ethnographic research through grounded theory practice. In: A. Bryant and K. Charmaz (eds), *Handbook of Grounded Theory*, London: Sage. pp. 493–513.

Tomlin, Z., Donovan, J. and Dieppe, P. (2007). Opening the black box of equipoise in randomised controlled trials. Presentation at BSA Medical Sociology Conference, Liverpool, September 2007.

Torgerson, D.J. (1998). Understanding controlled trials: what are pragmatic trials? *British Medical Journal*, 319: 285.

Torgerson, D.J., Klaber-Moffett, J. and Russell, I.T. (1996). Patient preferences in randomised trials: threat or opportunity? *Journal of Health Services Research and Policy*, 1(4):194–7.

Toynbee, P. (2006). Attacks on the decisions over the value of drugs are being used as a battering ram to break support for the NHS. *The Guardian*, 24 October 2006.

Traynor, M. (2009). Indeterminacy and technicality revisited: how medicine and nursing have responded to the evidence based movement. *Sociology of Health and Illness*, 31(4): 494–507.

Tunis, S.R. (2003). Practical clinical trials: increasing the value of clinical research. *Journal of the American Medical Association*, 290: 1634–2.

Turner, E.H., et al., (2008). Selective publication of antidepressant trials and its influence on apparent efficacy. *New England Journal of Medicine*, 358(3): 252–60.

UK Clinical Research Collaboration (2010). *UK Clinical Research Collaboration.* http://www.ukcrc.org/. [Accessed February 2010].

Vailly, J. (2006). Genetic screening as a technique of government: The case of neonatal screening for cystic fibrosis in France. *Social Science & Medicine*, 63(12): 3092–101.

Wager, E., Tooley, P.J.H. et al. (1995). How to do it: Get patients' consent to enter clinical trials. *British Medical Journal*, 311: 734–42.

Watson, E., Jenkins, L., Bukach, C. and Austoker, J. (2002). *The PSA Ttest and Prostate Cancer: Information for Primary Care.* NHS Cancer Screening Programmes: Sheffield, <http://www.cancerscreening.nhs.uk/prostate/> [Accessed July 2007]

Webster, A. (2007). Reflections on reflexive engagement. Response to Nowotny and Wynne. *Science, Technology and Human Values*, 32(5): 608–15.

Weinstein, M.C. and Stason, W.B. (1977). Foundations of cost-effectiveness analysis for health and medical practices. *New England Journal of Medicine*, 296: 716–21.

Wilkinson, R.G. and Pickett, K.G. (2009). *The Spirit Level. Why More Equal Societies Almost Always do Better.* London: Allen Lane.

Will, C. (2007). The alchemy of clinical trials. *Biosocieties*, Special Issue, 2(1): 85–99.

Will, C. (2009). Identifying effectiveness in "the old old": principles and values in the age of clinical trials. *Science, Technology and Human Values*, 34: 607–28.

Williams, I., McIver, S., Moore, D. and Bryan, S. (2008). The use of economic evaluations in NHS decision-making: a review and empirical investigation. *Health Technology Assessment*, 12: iii, ix–x, 1–175.

Williams, T., May, C., Mair, F., Mort, M. and Gask, L. (2003). Normative models of health technology assessment and the social production of evidence about telehealth care. *Health Policy*, 64(1): 39–54.

Winslow, B.T., Voorhees, K.I. and Pehl, K.A. (2007). Methamphetamine abuse. *American Family Physician*, 76(8): 1169–74.

Winterton, R. (2006). Written Answers to Questions [17 Mar 2006] – Prostate Cancer. Hansard Volume No. 443 Part No. 127. http://www.publications. parliament.uk/pa/cm200506/cmhansrd/vo060317/text/60317w17. htm#60317w17.html_spnew5. [Accessed June 2008].

Wood, M., Ferlie, E. and Fitzgerald, L. (1999). Achieving clinical behaviour change: a case of becoming indeterminate. *Social Sciences and Medicine*, 47(11): 1720–38.

World Health Organisation. (1982). *Manual on Environmental Management for Mosquito Control, with Special Emphasis on Malaria Vectors.* WHO Offset Publication No. 66, World Health Organisation.

World Health Organisation. (2002). *Safety of Medicines. A Guide to Detecting and Reporting Adverse Drug Reactions. Why Health Professionals Need to Take Action.* Geneva: World Health Organisation. Available at http://whqlibdoc. who.int/hq/2002/WHO_EDM_QSM_2002.2.pdf [accessed 8 March 2010].

Worrall, J. (2002). What evidence in evidence-based medicine. *Philosophy of Science*, 69: S316–S330.

Wozniak, P. (2003). Correspondence: Statin Wars. *The Lancet*, 363: 1855.

Wright, D., Sathe, N. and Spagnola, K. (2007). *State Estimates of Substance Use from the 2004–2005 National Surveys on Drug Use and Health.* Rockville, MD: Office of Applied Studies.

Yusuf, S., Lonn, E. and Bosch, J. (2009). Lipid lowering for primary prevention. *The Lancet*, 373: 1151–55.

Zorgverzekeraars Nederland en GGZ Nederland, (2008). In- en Verkoopgids DBC GGZ 2009 [Netherlands Health Insurers and Mental Health Organisations, 2008. Acquisition and Sales Guide of Diagnosis-Treatment Combinations in Mental Health 2009]. Zeist/Amersfoort: Zorgverzekeraars Nederland and GGZ Nederland. Available at www.zn.nl/leeszaal/zn_uitgaven/znuitgaven/in_ en_verkoopgids_dbc_ggz_2009.asp [accessed 30 March 2010].

Index

For Product Safety Concerns and Information please contact our EU
representative GPSR@taylorandfrancis.com
Taylor & Francis Verlag GmbH, Kaufingerstraße 24, 80331 München, Germany

www.ingramcontent.com/pod-product-compliance
Lightning Source LLC
Chambersburg PA
CBHW070717220326
41598CB00024BA/3199